STUDY BOOSTER FOR OET

Reading, Writing and Speaking skills development for effective communication in healthcare settings

BETH MCNALLY AND ANNE MACKENZIE

Study Booster for OET

Reading, Writing and Speaking skills development for effective communication in healthcare settings

Beth McNally and Anne Mackenzie

Copyright © 2022 B.McNally and A.Mackenzie. All rights reserved. Except for the quotation of short passages for the purposes of criticism and review, no part of this publication may be reproduced, stored in a retrieval system, or transmitted in any form or by any means, electronic, mechanical, photocopying, recording, or otherwise, without the prior written permission of the Copyright Authority Ltd. or the authors.

ISBN number:	ISBN 978-0-6482043-1-2
Cover & text design:	Dionne Del Rae

Disclaimer

Although the authors have made every effort to ensure that the information in this book was correct at press time, the authors do not assume and hereby disclaim any liability to any party for any loss, damage, or disruption caused by errors or omissions, whether such errors or omissions result from negligence, accident, or any other cause.

CONTENTS

INTRODUCTION		**IV**
UNIT 1	**FRACTURE CARE**	**1**
UNIT 2	**ALLERGY SYMPTOM RELIEF**	**15**
UNIT 3	**DIABETES MANAGEMENT**	**29**
UNIT 4	**FOCUS ON COMMON ERRORS 1: SPELLING**	**45**
UNIT 5	**CONSOLIDATION 1: UNITS 1-4**	**51**
UNIT 6	**GASTROINTESTINAL INVESTIGATIONS**	**61**
UNIT 7	**INFECTION PREVENTION AND CONTROL**	**77**
UNIT 8	**MEDICAL EMERGENCIES**	**97**
UNIT 9	**FOCUS ON COMMON ERRORS 2: FORMAL AND INFORMAL LANGUAGE**	**125**
UNIT 10	**CONSOLIDATION 2: UNITS 6-9**	**135**
ANSWER KEY	**UNITS 1-10**	**149**

MAP OF THE BOOK

UNITS 1-5

UNIT	UNIT NAME	READING	WRITING	SPEAKING
1	FRACTURE CARE	Identifying main ideas and locating specific information		Establishing and building rapport in patient-centred care
2	ALLERGY SYMPTOM RELIEF	Identifying main ideas and locating specific information	Using capital letters in medical correspondence	
3	DIABETES MANAGEMENT	Identifying main ideas and locating specific information		Identifying, acknowledging and incorporating the patient's perspective
4	FOCUS ON COMMON ERRORS 1: Spelling		Using accurate and standardised spelling in medical documentation	
5	CONSOLIDATION 1: Units 1-4	Review: Identifying main ideas and locating specific information	Review: Using capital letters and spelling in medical correspondence	Review: Establishing and building rapport in patient-centred care Identifying, acknowledging and incorporating the patient's perspective

MAP OF THE BOOK

UNITS 6-10

UNIT	UNIT NAME	READING	WRITING	SPEAKING
6	GASTROINTESTINAL INVESTIGATIONS	Identifying main ideas and locating specific information	Organising a medical letter	
7	INFECTION PREVENTION AND CONTROL	Recognising attitude, opinion and pronoun references		Managing the structure of discourse in a consultation Using cohesive devices
8	MEDICAL EMERGENCIES	Recognising attitude, opinion and pronoun references	Selecting and transforming case notes	
9	FOCUS ON COMMON ERRORS 2: Formal and informal language		Identifying appropriate language style in written healthcare contexts	Identifying appropriate language style in spoken healthcare contexts
10	CONSOLIDATION 2: Units 6-9	Review: Identifying main ideas and locating specific information Recognising attitude, opinion and pronoun references	Review: Organising a medical letter Selecting and transforming case notes Identifying and using appropriate language in written healthcare contexts	Review: Managing the structure of discourse in a consultation Identifying and using appropriate language in spoken healthcare contexts

INTRODUCTION

Study Booster for OET has been designed to support healthcare professionals seeking to boost their English language proficiency through increased awareness of Reading, Writing and Speaking skills presented and practised in a range of healthcare settings.

WHO IS THIS BOOK FOR?

Study Booster for OET is most suitable for healthcare professionals who:
- have a current minimum English language proficiency of CEFR B2+/C1.
- plan to have their English language proficiency assessed through the Occupational English Test (OET).

WHAT IS THE AIM OF THIS BOOK?

Study Booster for OET aims to identify and develop reading, writing and speaking skills in a range of healthcare settings. It is a user-friendly resource which provides relevant practice tasks devised to promote awareness and confidence in using:

Reading strategies to become powerful readers able to identify gist, locate specific information and interpret opinion and pronoun references.

Writing structures to become clear, precise writers of medical correspondence, including Letters of Discharge, Transfer and Referral.

Speaking rubric and sentence constructs to become effective and versatile communicators, displaying empathy, establishing rapport and structuring discourse to engage listeners.

Study Booster for OET can be used for independent study or integrated into a specialised course curriculum to consolidate Reading, Writing and Speaking skills development in English language healthcare-related courses, including English for Academic Purposes (EAP) for Nursing/Medicine and OET preparation courses.

It should be noted that while *Study Booster for OET* is a valuable supplementary Reading, Writing and Speaking skills development resource for healthcare students and professionals preparing for the OET, it is neither a dedicated OET preparation course, nor a medical textbook.

HOW IS THIS BOOK ORGANISED?

Study Booster for OET comprises ten stand-alone units which offer flexibility for the independent learner to select and focus on individual skill areas requiring development. The classroom or online teacher may also select appropriate units or particular skill booster tasks within a unit to supplement core teaching resources and address common areas of difficulty.

Units 1-3 and 6-8 feature:
- Reading skills with vocabulary development.
- Writing or Speaking skills development.
- practice tasks to develop proficiency in applying the skills to healthcare contexts.

Units 4 and 9 feature:
- frequently-occurring errors that have been identified as causing confusion for learners.
- practice tasks to develop strategies for accurate and appropriate language usage in medical correspondence and spoken interaction.

Units 5 and 10 are:
- Consolidation units designed to recycle and practise essential Reading, Writing and Speaking skill areas explored in Units 1-4 and 6-9.

WHO ARE THE AUTHORS?

The authors are English language specialists who have combined their English language knowledge and teaching and assessment experience to develop a valuable skill development resource, which focuses on the understanding and practice of Reading, Writing and Speaking in specific healthcare contexts.

The authors have written *Study Booster for OET* in consultation with healthcare professionals to ensure the accuracy and relevance of the content and terminology in the healthcare scenarios presented in the book.

Beth McNally: Beth has extensive experience of teaching and assessing courses in internationally-recognised English examination preparation and teacher training. It was while she was developing and teaching an English language course for Diploma of Nursing students (English for Nurses) that she first saw the need for English language resources specifically designed for healthcare professionals.

Anne Mackenzie: Anne has a wide-ranging career as an English language teacher, assessor, curriculum designer and education consultant in Australia, the Middle East, Asia and the UK. Anne has developed curriculum for a broad scope of English language courses, including internationally-recognised examination preparation and English for Academic Purposes for Nursing.

Grammar Booster for OET Nursing

Beth and Anne are the co-authors of the very successful *Grammar Booster for OET* Nursing, a resource designed to enhance language proficiency and effective communication in healthcare settings. Recognising an equally important need for a specific Reading, Writing and Speaking skills resource for healthcare professionals aiming to increase their English language skill proficiency, Beth and Anne collaborated to produce *Study Booster for OET*.

Both *Grammar Booster for OET Nursing* and *Study Booster for OET* can be used separately as independent resources or as complementary resources.

UNIT 1   FRACTURE CARE

STUDY FOCUS

Reading: Identifying main ideas and locating specific information

Vocabulary: Exploring fracture care and risks to bone health

Speaking: Establishing and building rapport in patient-centred care

Exploring the topic

In pairs or groups, discuss the following questions.

- What is the difference between a sprain, a dislocation and a fracture?
- What are possible causes of these injuries?
- Have you ever treated a fracture? What did the treatment involve?

STUDY BOOST 1: READING AND VOCABULARY

READING 1

Read the text and choose the most suitable heading A, B or C. Put a tick (✔) in the space provided at the end of the line.

> **BOOSTER TIP**
>
> For this task, read quickly to identify the **main idea** of the text. You do not need to focus on all of the information given.

A   Possible complications of bone fractures   _____

B   Clinical assessment of bone fractures   _____

C   First aid for bone fractures   _____

- Keep the injured person still, especially in the case of suspected skull, spinal, rib, pelvic or upper leg fracture.
- Apply direct pressure using a clean dressing to control external haemorrhage.
- Immobilise the affected area by applying a splint or sling if available.
- Provide pain relief if needed.
- Apply an ice pack to the injured area to reduce swelling and pain.
- Where the injury is to a limb, elevate using a sling for arm injuries, a pillow for leg injuries.
- If in doubt, always treat the injury as a fracture.
- Do not attempt to realign broken bones.
- An open fracture (where the bone is visible) is considered a medical emergency. Seek medical assistance urgently.

VOCABULARY PRACTICE 1: SENTENCE COMPLETION

Read the text again and use the words in the box to complete the sentences. There is one extra word that you do not need to use. An example (0) has been done for you.

| straighten | bleeding | minimise | unsure | call |
| contact | ~~ensure~~ | administer | raise | still |

0 **Ensure** the injured person does not move.

1 Use direct pressure to stop any external _____.

2 A sling or splint is recommended to keep the affected area _____.

3 _____ pain relief to patients who are in severe pain.

4 _____ swelling with the application of an ice pack.

5 If possible, use a pillow to _____ the injured leg.

6 If you are _____ about an injury, treat it as a fracture.

7 Never try to _____ a broken bone by forcing it back into place.

8 If you can see the broken bone, _____ for emergency assistance.

READING 2

Task 1

Read the text about fracture risk and bone health and choose the most suitable answer A, B or C. Put a tick (✔) in the space provided at the end of the line.

> **BOOSTER TIP**
>
> For this task, read quickly to identify the **purpose** of the text. You do not need to focus on all of the information given.

The purpose of this text is to

A explain the benefits of bone mineral density testing.   _____

B report on major contributory causes of fracture.   _____

C argue against lifestyle changes to minimise fracture risk.   _____

Fracture risk and bone health

Fractures are common in children and are often the result of a traumatic incident such as a fall or a sporting injury. As bones continue to grow throughout childhood, they are more flexible, but also more fragile than fully developed adult bones. The wrist, arm and elbow are the most frequently seen fracture sites in children. Bones reach their maximum strength and density (peak bone mass) somewhere between late adolescence and the early thirties, after which bones progressively lose minerals, mass and structure.

Several factors are known to adversely affect bone health and increase the risk of fracture, including age, sex, disease and lifestyle. With advancing age, bones weaken and are increasingly prone to fracture. Women have a higher risk of fracture than men due to the rapid decline in oestrogen levels during menopause, which causes bones to break down more quickly.

Certain diseases can also cause bones to become brittle and vulnerable to fracture, with osteoporosis being perhaps the best-known example. Osteoporosis is characterised by low bone mineral density and usually causes no symptoms. People who have this disease are often unaware until a fracture occurs. Osteoporosis can cause bone to fracture without significant trauma, by coughing, for example.

A bone density scan measures the concentration of calcium and other bone minerals in the sample section of bone and can identify osteoporosis. Many medical experts used to consider measurements of bone mineral density alone to be the strongest predictor of fracture risk. However, this is now known not to be the case. According to recent research, many people with an osteoporotic bone density never fracture, while many fractures occur in people whose bone density measurements fall within the normal range.

Bone density measurements are now considered in combination with other important indicators to evaluate fracture risk. Studies have shown low body weight, deficiencies in calcium and vitamins D and K and a high rate of bone resorption to be stronger fracture predictors than bone density alone.

Lifestyle choices including smoking, alcohol consumption and exercise also play a significant role in bone health. Tobacco use is associated with decreased bone density and increased risk of fracture while consuming more than three alcoholic beverages per day affects the metabolism of vitamin D and depletes calcium reserves. Avoiding a sedentary lifestyle by participating in regular physical activity, including weight-bearing exercise, is vital for maintaining bone density.

Task 2

Read the text again. Answer Questions 1-5 with a word or short phrase from the text. An example (0) has been done for you.

> **BOOSTER TIP**
>
> For this task, read the text carefully to locate the **specific information** required for each question. Read the details closely to ensure clear understanding of the text and questions.

Questions 1-5

0 What are two common causes of fracture in children?
<u>**a fall, a sporting injury**</u>

1 Which three parts of the body are the most frequently fractured in children?
_____

2 What commonly leads to bone density loss in women as they age?
_____

3 In the past, what was thought to be the best indicator of fracture risk?
_____

4 A lack of which vitamins and minerals can contribute to fracture risk?
_____

5 What specific type of exercise should be performed regularly to maintain bone health?
_____

Questions 6-10

For Questions 6-10, decide whether the statements are true (T) or false (F).

6	Peak bone mass occurs prior to the teenage years.	T	F
7	Men are more likely to experience a fracture than women.	T	F
8	Osteoporotic bones can fracture as a result of minor trauma to the bone.	T	F
9	Fractures commonly occur in people with no evidence of decreased bone density.	T	F
10	Everyday habits have no impact on bone health.	T	F

VOCABULARY PRACTICE 2A: MATCHING MEANING

The words and phrases in Column A appear in Reading 2. Choose the most suitable word or phrase from Column B for each word or phrase in Column A. Write your answers in the space provided. An example (0) has been done for you.

COLUMN A		COLUMN B	
0	fragile	A	inactive, stationary
1	adolescence	B	linked to
2	minerals	C	not enough of something
3	adversely	D	for example, calcium, iron, zinc
4	significant	E	susceptible to/likely to
5	deficiency	F	the period of development between childhood and adulthood
6	associated with	G	to reduce the amount of something
7	deplete	H	negatively
8	reserves	I	frail, weak, not strong
9	sedentary	J	important
10	prone to	K	a supply of something that is kept until it is needed

Write your answers here.

0	1	2	3	4	5	6	7	8	9	10
I										

VOCABULARY PRACTICE 2B: COMPLETE THE SENTENCE

Choose the most suitable word or phrase from the box to complete each sentence. An example (0) has been done for you.

mineral	adolescence	deficiency	associated with	prone to
sedentary	reserves	significant	fragile	depletes	adversely

0   Health professionals advise against a **sedentary** lifestyle which may lead to poor health outcomes.

1   Bones during _____ are generally less _____ than in childhood.

2   Children and adults (aged 65+) are more _____ fracture than young adults.

3   When calcium intake is low, the body uses its _____ of calcium in the bone.
    This _____ stored calcium and results in the loss of bone _____ density.

4   Leading an active life and eating a healthy diet are _____ good bone health.

5   Recent studies have found that a _____ in calcium can _____ affect bone health and may lead to a _____ increase in osteoporosis risk.

READING 3

Read the text about post-fracture physiotherapy interventions for improving upper and lower limb function. For Questions 1-6, choose the most suitable answer A, B or C. An example (0) has been done for you.

BOOSTER TIP

For this task, read the text carefully to locate the **specific information** required for each question. Read the details closely to ensure clear understanding of the text and questions.

Post-fracture physiotherapy interventions for improving upper and lower limb function

Physiotherapists aim to optimise healing and the return to normal function of affected joints and muscles following a fracture. They use a variety of treatments, including manual physical therapy techniques, ultrasound or electrical stimulation, hydrotherapy, heat and ice to assist with pain management and rehabilitation.

Fractured bones generally require immobilisation with a cast or, in more complicated cases, with surgically inserted metal rods or plates, to hold the bone pieces together, ensuring alignment and healing in the correct position. While limbs are immobilised, however, their lack of use can result in decreased muscle tone and atrophy of the muscle.

Physiotherapists assess the impact of the fracture on the functionality of the affected limb in order to develop customised treatment plans for each patient which will assist with restoring muscle strength and preventing secondary complications.

Physiotherapists also provide the patient with practical support throughout treatment and recovery. For fractures involving a cast, the physiotherapist will advise patients to keep the injured limb elevated as much as possible. After the cast has been applied, patients should exercise fingers or toes of the affected limb as often as is bearable, particularly during the first 24 to 72 hours. This is to improve circulation, reduce swelling and to help prevent post-fracture stiffness and muscle weakness.

If a fracture to the arm or shoulder requires the arm to be placed in a sling, the physiotherapist will train patients to apply and remove the sling and will provide instruction in activities that focus on reaching for and grasping objects.

Following a fracture to the leg, the physiotherapist will recommend the most suitable walking aid, such as a rollator, wheelie walker, crutches or a cane to support mobility while the bone is healing. The physiotherapist will guide and monitor patients as they learn how to safely move around their environment, including walking up and down stairs, sitting and standing from a chair and getting in and out of a car.

Physiotherapists introduce the patient to specialised exercises which focus on improving balance, range of motion, strength and function. In order for patients to participate as comfortably as possible without experiencing further exercise-related pain, physiotherapists generally recommend that prescribed pain relief medication is taken between 30 minutes and one hour prior to starting the physical treatment sessions.

Balance exercises should be practised daily. These exercises help the patient to develop control over their body when maintaining a stationary position, for example, when balancing on one leg (static balance) and also whenever they are moving (dynamic balance). If static balance is impaired, the likelihood of patients falling is much greater. Without good dynamic balance, patients may not be able to adapt to different positions and maintain their centre of gravity, which may result in back pain, hip pain or knee pain.

Range of motion exercises increase the ability to move a joint from fully flexed to fully extended and are vital to the recovery process. The physiotherapist will decide which range of motion exercises are suitable for each patient. If the patient is unable to move the limb independently, the physiotherapist will move the limb for the patient through a range of passive motion exercises.

As recovery progresses and the affected muscles are healing, the patient will commence strengthening active-assistance exercises, receiving partial support from the physiotherapist to move the limb until the patient's pain threshold is reached.

Once the fracture has healed and the patient is well on the way to regaining optimal functionality, the physiotherapist will devise a program of active exercises which can be completed without assistance.

Questions 1-6

0 A fracture can be immobilised with

    A   a rollator

    B   a cane.

    C   **a cast.**

1   Immobilising a broken bone is done

    A   to decrease swelling.

    B   to reposition the bone correctly.

    C   to prevent muscle shrinkage.

2   Physiotherapist guidelines for a fracture in the first three days after a cast has set include

    A   stretching neck and back muscles.

    B   stretching fingers and toes ten times per day.

    C   maintaining the injured area in a raised position.

3   If an upper limb has been fractured, the physiotherapist will help the patient to learn

    A   how to pick up and hold everyday items.

    B   how to use crutches.

    C   how to walk independently.

4 Taking prescribed pain relief medication before physical therapy is recommended
   A to reduce swelling.
   B to minimise uncontrolled pain when moving the injured limb.
   C to be able to balance on one leg.

5 Balance exercises
   A may cause a patient to experience back pain.
   B should be performed weekly.
   C may reduce the risk of a patient falling.

6 Passive motion exercises are designed for patients who
   A can complete them unassisted.
   B need assistance to complete them.
   C have regained full functionality of the injured limb.

VOCABULARY PRACTICE 3: COMPLETE THE SENTENCE

For Questions 1-6, choose the most suitable answer A, B or C to complete each sentence. An example (0) has been done for you.

0 Physiotherapy is recommended after a fracture to restore _____ of the injured limb.
   A functional   **B functionality**   C functioning

1 Your physiotherapist will _____ you in correct techniques to practise the exercises.
   A instructions   B instructed   C instruct

2 You are advised to use a mobility aid if you are unable to move around _____ .
   A unassisted   B assistance   C assisted

3 The _____ program is selected by the physiotherapist in consultation with the patient.
   A untreated   B treated   C treatment

4 Ice is recommended to reduce _____ soft tissue around the fracture site.
   A swelled   B swollen   C swell

5 Electrical stimulation and ultrasound are recognised for their _____ value in accelerating bone healing.
   A therapeutic   B therapy   C therapist

6 An _____ stay in hospital is not required if healing is progressing satisfactorily.
   A extension   B extend   C extended

Discussion

1 What are common causes of fracture?
2 What factors contribute to declining bone health as we age?
3 What steps can be taken to maintain good bone health?
4 How can a physiotherapist assist the patient with regaining optimal functionality after a fracture?

STUDY BOOST 2: SPEAKING

Establishing and building rapport in patient-centred care

Establishing and building rapport during consultations can assist the healthcare professional to develop and maintain a supportive and collaborative relationship with a patient.

This involves showing empathy through responding with sensitivity to the patient's feelings and to their particular situation.

Communication strategies to establish and build rapport

We use both verbal and non-verbal techniques to establish and build rapport.

Effective verbal communication strategies include:

- **Using phrases and extra words to soften the language**

✔ It might be a good idea for your son to see a speech pathologist about his stutter. He is rather difficult to understand at times.

✘ Your son needs help from a speech pathologist. No-one can understand him.

✔ Your cat has a life-threatening condition, I'm afraid. We recommend surgery as soon as possible.

✘ Your cat needs surgery or she will die.

✔ I'm sorry but I don't have time to shower you now. I'll be able to do it later today.

✘ I can't shower you now. You'll have to wait.

- **Avoiding criticising the patient**

✔ You have quite a lot of plaque build-up. I'll remove it and then we'll take a look at how you brush your teeth.

✘ Your teeth are covered in plaque. You are obviously not brushing well enough.

✔ It's best not to use the Internet for medical advice. Please talk to a medical professional about your concerns.

✘ You should never rely on the Internet for medical advice.

✔ I can see fatty deposits on your liver. Your doctor will discuss that further with you.

✘ I can see fatty deposits on your liver. Your diet must be very unhealthy.

- **Choosing neutral language to avoid sounding judgemental**

✔ Here is a list of alternatives to soft drink for you to try.

✘ You drink far too much soft drink. You need to change that.

- ✔ Can I recommend some shoes which will support your feet better?
- ✘ These are cheap shoes, aren't they? It's no wonder you've developed bunions.

- ✔ It would be a good idea to consider not smoking while you are pregnant.
- ✘ You are pregnant! I can't believe you haven't stopped smoking.

- **Showing empathy**

- ✔ I realise that it may be difficult at first, but taking up regular exercise will improve your quality of life.
- ✘ You must start exercising regularly. It's not that hard.

- ✔ I understand that you would like your father to recuperate at home, but he needs specialist care.
- ✘ Your father cannot recuperate at home. You don't know how to care for him properly.

- ✔ You have thyroid cancer. I know it is a shock. I wish I had better news for you.
- ✘ You have thyroid cancer. When can we book you in for surgery?

- **Giving reassurance**

- ✔ You look quite worried. What can I do to help?
- ✘ There is nothing to worry about. We don't need to talk about this any more.

- ✔ Come back and see me again or call the clinic if you are concerned for any reason.
- ✘ There is no need to come back.

- ✔ Your wife is receiving the best care possible. We are doing everything we can.
- ✘ This clinic is the best in the region. Your wife has nothing to complain about.

> NOTE: **Non-verbal techniques** include actively listening to the patient, making eye contact and using appropriate body language, for example, nodding your head in agreement to show understanding when the patient is speaking.

SPEAKING PRACTICE 1: MULTIPLE CHOICE

A patient has presented to a medical clinic in significant pain with a bruised and swollen arm while on holidays. You suspect a fracture. Read the following patient comments and descriptions of their behaviour and the healthcare professional's responses. Choose the most suitable answer A or B. An example (0) has been done for you.

0 I want to see the doctor. NOW!

    A You have to wait your turn for the doctor. You are not an urgent case.

    B <u>I understand you want to see the doctor as soon as possible. I will let you know when the doctor is on the way.</u>

1. **Ow!! It hurts!**

   A   I know it hurts at the moment. We are doing everything possible to make you feel more comfortable.

   B   It is a very minor injury. You are overreacting.

2. **Patient is crying.**

   A   Why are you crying? Stop it. There is no need to cry.

   B   Here are some tissues. I know it is upsetting.

3. **Do not touch my arm.**

   A   I have to touch your arm to put the sling on.

   B   I will tell you when I need to touch your arm. I will be as gentle as possible.

4. **The painkillers are not working. It still hurts.**

   A   The pain relief will take effect very soon and you should start to feel more comfortable. I'll check on you again in a few minutes.

   B   I just administered it. You need to wait for it to work.

5. **My holiday is ruined!**

   A   Oh! That is really bad luck.

   B   Oh, well. It could be much worse.

6. **It's my own fault. I was skiing too fast.**

   A   Yes, you were. You should have been more careful.

   B   Lots of people fall. You were just unlucky, unfortunately.

7. **Could you please wait with me until the doctor arrives?**

   A   Sorry, no. I have other patients to look after.

   B   I'll check on you again soon. I can put the TV on for you and give you a couple of magazines to read.

8. **Why can't you get in contact with my partner?**

   A   I have not had time. You will have to wait until the end of my shift.

   B   I have tried the number you gave me, but there was no answer. Do you have a different number that I can call?

9. **I hope I can go home today.**

   A   No, it's not possible.

   B   I understand, but unfortunately you need to stay in hospital for a few more days.

10. **I'm hungry.**

    A   I'm so sorry, but you can't have anything to eat until we know if you need surgery.

    B   You can't eat now.

SPEAKING PRACTICE 2: WHAT WOULD YOU SAY?

What would you say to show empathy to people in the following situations?

1 a patient with coeliac disease who needs to eliminate gluten from their diet
2 the owner of a seriously ill dog which has contracted a virus
3 a teenager who needs braces and is worried about their appearance
4 a patient who has developed an eye infection because they have not been cleaning their contact lenses properly
5 a patient whose ultrasound has detected an abnormally enlarged spleen
6 an exhausted new mother who is having trouble breastfeeding

SPEAKING PRACTICE 3: ROLE PLAY

ROLE PLAY 1

Work in pairs as healthcare professional and patient. Read your role play card to familiarise yourself with the task. Take a few minutes to plan what you are going to say. You can make notes during the preparation time if you wish.

BOOSTER TIP
For this task, demonstrate that you have established and built rapport with the patient.

ROLE PLAY 1

ROLE A: HEALTHCARE PROFESSIONAL   **SETTING: ALPINE MEDICAL CLINIC**

A patient presents with a suspected distal radius (wrist) fracture after falling while skiing. He/she is frustrated about the need for a cast because he/she works as a piano teacher. He/she is upset about being injured while on holiday.

TASK

- Enquire whether the patient has pain, bruising or swelling.

- Inform the patient that you are going to elevate the affected area using a pillow for support.

- When asked, explain the importance of elevation at the level of the heart to help decrease swelling and pain.

- Explain the process of diagnosing a fracture, including examination by a doctor, imaging, possible surgery and the need for a cast.

- Emphasise that a cast will help the fracture to heal correctly. Mention the benefits of a fibreglass cast (a lighter, synthetic alternative to a traditional plaster cast).

- Inform the patient that the cast is usually worn for around 6 weeks. A removable splint will be used to support the wrist after the cast has been removed.

- Reassure the patient that with the proper treatment the prognosis is good. Recommend follow-up with an occupational therapist to support rehabilitation.

- Be understanding of the patient's feelings that their holiday has been ruined.

ROLE PLAY 1

ROLE B: PATIENT   **SETTING: ALPINE MEDICAL CLINIC**

You have been brought to the medical clinic by ski patrol after falling on your wrist while skiing. You are distressed about the need for a cast because you believe it will affect your job as a piano teacher. You are upset that you have been injured while on holiday.

TASK

- When asked, tell the healthcare professional you have severe pain in your wrist. It feels tender and is swollen.
- Ask why your wrist needs to be elevated.
- Ask the healthcare professional to explain the procedure for treating a fracture.
- Appear distressed about having to wear a cast as your hands are essential to your job as a piano teacher.
- Ask how long it will be necessary to wear a cast.
- Admit that you are concerned about long-term problems with your wrist.
- Tell the healthcare professional that you feel upset that your holiday has been ruined.

ROLE PLAY 2

Work in pairs as healthcare professional and patient. Read your role play card to familiarise yourself with the task. Take a few minutes to plan what you are going to say. You can make notes during the preparation time if you wish.

ROLE PLAY 2

ROLE A: HEALTHCARE PROFESSIONAL **SETTING: SNOWY MOUNTAIN HOSPITAL**

Your patient has had surgery to stabilise a fractured tibia and fibula sustained while snowboarding. The patient is now recovering on the ward.

TASK

- Ask if the patient is experiencing any pain.
- Explain to the patient that they have had the maximum amount of pain relief and more pain relief will be offered in 4 hours' time.
- Suggest other ways of managing the pain, such as elevating the limb, applying an ice pack and using deep breathing techniques.
- When asked, explain that the plates and screws will stabilise the ankle joint and allow the bones to heal correctly.
- If asked, explain that the risk of infection is relatively low, and intravenous antibiotics were administered during surgery to help prevent infection.
- Emphasise the importance of physiotherapy to support recovery and restore full range of motion.
- Inform the patient that he/she will not be able to drive for 2-4 weeks.
- Reassure the patient that you expect him/her to make a full recovery.

ROLE PLAY 2

ROLE B: PATIENT   **SETTING: SNOWY MOUNTAIN HOSPITAL**

You fractured your ankle while snowboarding on holiday. The injury required surgery to stabilise the bones in your ankle using plates and screws. You are recovering on the ward.

TASK

- When asked, tell the healthcare professional you are in a significant amount of pain.

- Appear agitated when you are told you need to wait 4 hours before you receive more pain relief Tell the healthcare professional that you feel he/she does not understand the amount of pain you are in.

- Ask the healthcare professional to explain why you needed plates and screws in your ankle.

- Tell the healthcare professional that you are worried about developing an infection.

- Ask if you will need physiotherapy.

- Appear annoyed that you will not be able to drive for several weeks.

UNIT 2   ALLERGY SYMPTOM RELIEF

STUDY FOCUS

Reading: Identifying main ideas and locating specific information
Vocabulary: Managing symptoms of allergic reactions
Writing: Using capital letters in medical correspondence

Exploring the topic

In pairs or groups, discuss the following questions.

- What are some common symptoms of allergies?
- What can allergy sufferers do to ease their symptoms?
- What are some examples of allergens in the environment?

STUDY BOOST 1: READING AND VOCABULARY

READING 1

Task 1

Choose the heading, A, B or C, which best describes the main idea of Reading 1. Put a tick (✔) in the space provided at the end of the line.

BOOSTER TIP

For this task, read quickly to identify the **main idea** of the text. You do not need to focus on all of the information given.

A   Various allergens encountered in the environment   _____
B   A specific allergen commonly found indoors   _____
C   Symptoms of environmental allergies   _____

House dust mites are ubiquitous in our environment. They are microscopic beings and are therefore invisible to the naked eye. Dust mites feed off skin flakes that are continuously shed by humans. People who are allergic to dust mites are actually allergic to the antigen that is present in the mite faeces. This antigen can contribute to asthma, eczema and allergic rhinitis. Patients who suffer from asthma, eczema or allergic rhinitis and are allergic to the house dust mite allergen can benefit from reduced exposure to the dust mite allergen.

House dust mites cannot be eliminated from our surroundings. However, we can reduce the number of mites and the amount of allergen in our surroundings by modifying our home environment, particularly in the bedroom.

There are a number of environmental modifications that help to reduce exposure to the house dust mite allergen. Remove all soft toys and soft furnishings such as cushions from the bedroom as well as any woollen underlay from the bed. Wash all bedding in hot water (>55°C) weekly and dry it in full sunshine where possible or tumble dry on a hot setting. Vacuum carpet thoroughly and mop hard flooring on a weekly basis. Dust hard surfaces in the bedroom regularly with a damp cloth. Commercially available dust mite resistant covers are also recommended for pillows, quilts and mattresses.

Although many bedrooms have carpets or rugs on the floor which can trap dust mites and allergens, the removal of carpets is controversial and is generally not recommended as a first step to reduce the number of house mites and allergens until other options have been explored.

Dust mites living in carpets can be disturbed when people move about on the carpet. However, as dust mites are relatively heavy and fall rapidly following disturbance, instead of removing carpets, a more reasonable approach is to discourage sitting or lying on carpets and rugs. Since we spend up to 10 hours each day sleeping, it is better to focus on reducing the dust mite population on the bed rather than on carpets or rugs.

Air purifiers are designed to reduce pollutants floating in the air, including smoke, pollen and pet dander. Air purifiers are generally not recommended to reduce the accumulation of dust mites as the weight of the dust mites prevents them from remaining airborne for any length of time.

Allergy testing (including blood tests and skin prick tests) can determine whether house dust mites are triggering symptoms.

Task 2

Read the text again. For Questions 1-8, decide whether the statements are true (T) or false (F). An example (0) has been done for you.

Questions 1-8

0	House dust mites exist everywhere in our home environment.	**T**	F
1	House dust mites can be seen without a microscope.	T	F
2	Minimising exposure to the dust mite allergen can reduce certain symptoms for allergy sufferers.	T	F
3	Efforts to lower the number of dust mites should be mainly focused on the bedroom.	T	F
4	Bedding must be washed several times per week.	T	F
5	Experts agree that removing all carpets and rugs in bedrooms is necessary.	T	F
6	The dust mite allergen tends to remain in the air.	T	F
7	Air purifiers are not particularly useful for sufferers of dust mite allergies.	T	F
8	Dust mite allergies can be diagnosed through more than one type of test.	T	F

VOCABULARY PRACTICE 1: MATCHING MEANING

The words and phrases in Column A appear in Reading 1. Choose the most suitable word or phrase from Column B for each word or phrase in Column A. Write your answers in the space provided. An example (0) has been done for you.

COLUMN A		COLUMN B	
0	<u>ubiquitous</u>	A	to adapt or adjust
1	microscopic	B	<u>everywhere</u>
2	benefit	C	causes disagreement, discussion
3	eliminate	D	to gain something positive
4	modify	E	floating in the air
5	thoroughly	F	to remove, dispose of
6	weekly	G	completely, comprehensively
7	controversial	H	to cause, produce
8	airborne	I	once every seven days
9	relatively	J	extremely small, miniscule
10	trigger	K	comparatively

Write your answers here.

0	1	2	3	4	5	6	7	8	9	10
B										

READING 2

Read the following text about mucus. For Questions 1-5, choose the most suitable answer A, B or C. An example (0) has been done for you.

> **BOOSTER TIP**
>
> For this task, read the text carefully to locate the **specific information** required for each question. Read the details closely to ensure clear understanding of the text and questions.

Mucus

The antibacterial enzymes and proteins (antibodies) in mucus kill and trap germs, protecting us from infection. Allergies, environmental irritants and sickness can increase the production of mucus from nasal mucous membranes. Thicker mucus which accumulates in the back of the nose and throat and drains through the back of the nasal cavity is often referred to as postnasal drip. It may be caused by dry air, bacterial infections, dehydration or smoking and can cause a crust to form, leading to the production of bacteria. This interferes with normal nasal function of warming, filtering and humidifying air prior to it reaching the lungs. Throats become more sensitive, causing a cough.

Management and treatment of thicker mucus includes the use of saline (nasal rinsing), nasal decongestants, intranasal antihistamine and medicated nasal sprays.

Saline can help to control symptoms by thinning down the mucus in the nasal passages and flushing it out. This makes it easier to breathe through the nose and to swallow. The use of distilled, sterile or boiled water for saline nasal rinsing is recommended.

Nasal decongestants are available over the counter and provide rapid relief of symptoms. It should be noted, however, that prolonged use of nasal decongestants causes swelling in the nose and can result in more severe symptoms of congestion and headaches. This is called rebound congestion.

Intranasal antihistamines are nasal sprays which reduce nasal inflammation caused by allergic rhinitis (hayfever) and are generally considered to be first line therapy in hayfever treatment. However, intranasal corticosteroids provide greater relief for those with severe congestion.

Medicated nasal sprays (intranasal corticosteroids and intranasal antihistamine plus corticosteroids) are particularly useful for severe allergic rhinitis and can be more effective than oral antihistamines. This is due to the local anti-inflammatory effect these medications produce, reducing mucus production and relieving the symptoms associated with congestion, such as a blocked or runny nose, headaches and the feeling of pressure in your sinuses. They may be appropriate for the treatment of seasonal and perennial allergic rhinitis.

Questions 1-5

0   Mucus plays a role in
   A   **protecting the body from illness.**
   B   preventing allergies.
   C   maintaining hydration in the nasal passages.

1   Postnasal drip
   A   collects only in the throat.
   B   encourages the development of bacteria.
   C   improves the nasal function of warming air going to the lungs.

2   Nasal rinsing
   A   works best with untreated tap water.
   B   makes swallowing more challenging.
   C   increases the fluidity of mucus.

3   Long-term use of nasal decongestants is
   A   by prescription only.
   B   generally not recommended.
   C   most useful for those suffering congestion and headaches.

4   The initial treatment generally recommended for hayfever is
   A   an intranasal antihistamine.
   B   a medicated nasal spray.
   C   a nasal decongestant.

5   Medicated nasal sprays used to treat severe cases of allergic rhinitis
   A   are more cost-effective than other medications.
   B   may ease a number of symptoms.
   C   do not work as well as oral antihistamines alone.

VOCABULARY PRACTICE 2: WORD FORMS

Look carefully at each of the following sentences. Choose the most suitable option A, B or C to complete each sentence. An example (0) has been done for you.

0 He was prescribed a course of antibiotics to treat a bacterial _____.
  A infectious   **B infection**   C infected

1 Mr Baldwin was treated with medication to reduce _____ caused by an anaphylactic reaction.
  A swollen   B swelling   C swelled

2 Wearing _____ clothing such as gloves, gowns and masks in a hospital can help to prevent the spread of germs.
  A protective   B protection   C unprotected

3 Am I able to use a _____ to help clear my blocked nose?
  A decongestion   B decongested   C decongestant

4 Vomiting, diarrhoea, fever and sweating can all cause _____ in infants.
  A hydration   B dehydrated   C dehydration

5 How can I reduce eye, nose and throat _____ from indoor allergens?
  A irritation   B irritant   C irritable

READING 3

Read the following text about using a nasal spray. For Questions 1-5, choose the most suitable answer A, B or C. An example (0) has been done for you.

Step-by-step spray technique for patients

Priming the spray	Before using the spray for the first time, you need to prime the device by spraying several times into the air per the manufacturer's instructions until a fine mist appears. If you do not use your spray for several days, you will need to prime it again.
Getting prepared	1 Shake the bottle prior to each use. 2 If your nose is blocked by mucus, blow your nose gently. (If badly blocked, you may also need to rinse with saline before using the nasal spray. Wait 10 minutes after rinsing with saline before using a nasal spray.)
Before spraying	3 Tilt your head slightly forward. 4 Put the nozzle into one nostril using your opposite hand. (Right nostril, left hand.) 5 Close the other nostril using your free hand.

Spraying	6	Breathe in slowly and press to spray at the same time. Inhale the mist gently. Keep the mist inside the nose. Do not sniff hard during or immediately after spraying. Sniffing hard may cause the spray to bypass the nasal passage and force the mist into the back of the throat, where it may cause irritation or a burning sensation.
	7	Repeat steps 3-6 for the other nostril.
After spraying	8	Wipe the tip of the spray with a clean cloth and replace cap.
		If you are using two different nasal sprays wait 10 minutes before using the second spray.

Questions 1-5

0 Priming the device

    A must be done every day.

    B **makes it ready for use.**

    C releases heavy droplets of spray.

1 Immediately prior to using the spray, the user should
    A position their head to one side.
    B tilt their head backwards.
    C lean their head forward a little.

2 To clear a badly blocked nose, first blow the nose gently, and then
    A rinse the nose with saline and wait 10 minutes before using the nasal spray.
    B wait 10 minutes and rinse the nose with saline before using the nasal spray.
    C use the nasal spray and wait 10 minutes before rinsing the nose with saline.

3 If the nozzle is placed in the left nostril, according to the directions,
    A the device should be activated with the left hand.
    B the device should be activated with the right hand.
    C the device can be activated with either hand.

4 Sniffing hard directly after spraying may
    A direct the medication deep into the nasal passages.
    B irritate the nasal lining.
    C inflame the throat.

5 When using a nasal spray, users should
    A always clean the nozzle after use.
    B prime the device as directed for the first use only.
    C push the nozzle deep into the nose.

Discussion

1 How can nasal sprays help sufferers of allergic rhinitis?
2 How would you instruct a patient to use a nasal spray? What key information would you include in your explanation?
3 What general lifestyle advice would you give to an allergy sufferer?

STUDY BOOST 2: WRITING

Using capital letters in medical correspondence

It is important to know when to use capital letters. We use capital letters for:

The first letter of the first word in a sentence

Symptoms of atopic eczema include inflamed and itchy skin.

Your procedure has been booked for Wednesday, July 7 at 2pm.

The abbreviation Re: in the subject line of a letter

To introduce the subject of a letter, "Re:" meaning "regarding" is often used to state the reason for the letter, which includes a patient's personal details

Re: Ms Linda Reeves, aged 69

Re: Mr Jack Stone

DOB: 8 September 1968 *or* 08/09/68

36 Hall St

Cityside

Proper nouns

We always use a capital letter for the first letter of a proper noun. For example:

- **Titles and positions**

  Mr, **M**s, **M**rs, **M**iss, **D**r

  We use capital letters when referring to job titles and positions.

  We do NOT use capital letters when referring generally to a job or profession.

COMPARE:

Job titles	General reference to a job or profession
Fiona Lee, **L**actation **C**onsultant	The lactation consultant provided advice on feeding.
Dr Max Rowe, **E**ndodontist	Mr Wilson was referred to an endodontist.
Dr Remo Davi, **O**phthalmologist	Dr Remo Davi is an ophthalmologist.

- **First names, middle names, surnames**

  Timothy **J**oseph **R**obinson

  Ji **W**on **P**ark

  Stephanie **B**erson

- **Street names, city names, country names**

  Princess **S**treet

  Bologna

  India

- **Languages and nationalities**

  English

  Italian

  Japanese

  Spanish

- **Company names and names of institutions**
  City Orthopaedics
  Happy Pets Veterinary Surgery
  Mansfield Birth Centre
  Morningtown Medical Centre
  Smile Orthodontics
  St Patrick's Hospital

- **The personal pronoun**
  I

- **Days of the week, months of the year, public holidays and special days**
  Tuesday, Friday
  March, September
  Christmas Day
  Independence Day
  World Heart Day

- **The first word of a salutation**
  Dear Mr Watanabe

- **The first word of the complimentary close**
  Yours sincerely

- **Certain medical conditions, diseases or viruses which have been named after a person or place**
  Alzheimer's disease
  Crohn's disease
  Hodgkin lymphoma
  Turner's syndrome
  Ebola virus disease
  Zika virus disease

  > NOTE: We do NOT use capital letters to refer to viruses which do not contain the name of a person or place. For example:
  > adenovirus
  > cytomegalovirus

- **Names of species of bacteria**
  Escherichia coli bacteria *or* E. coli bacteria
  Salmonella bacteria
  Staphylococcus aureus bacteria *or* S. aureus bacteria

- **Medications**
  We use capital letters when referring to brands of medications.
  We do NOT use capital letters when referring to active ingredients of medications.

COMPARE:

Brands of medications	Active ingredients of medications
Panadol, Calpol, Tylenol	paracetamol
Zofran	ondansetron
Advil, Motrin	ibuprofen
Ventolin, Asmol	salbutamol
Nurofen Plus, Mersyndol	codeine
Nasonex	mometasone furoate
Zyrtec	cetirizine
Phenergan	promethazine

NOTE: We do NOT use capital letters to refer to common nouns including parts of the body, illnesses and names of procedures. For example:

adrenal gland	pericystitis	arthroplasty
pelvis	jaundice	biopsy
tendon	malaria	vaccination

WRITING PRACTICE 1: UNDERSTANDING AND USING CAPITAL LETTERS

Rewrite each phrase or sentence using capital letters where appropriate. An example (0) has been done for you.

0   thank you for seeing sean mulrooney in regard to his recent diagnosis of parkinson's disease.
    Thank you for seeing Sean Mulrooney in regard to his recent diagnosis of Parkinson's disease.

1   dear dr larkham
    _____

2   please present to the admissions desk at cityside hospital at 0800 on friday, august 12.
    _____

3   mr singh takes nasonex and zyrtec as needed.
    _____

4   mrs martin has been advised to take paracetamol (a maximum of 8 per day) to manage pain. her preference is to take panadol rather than a generic brand.
    _____
    _____

5   louisa shaw was born in boston, massachusetts in july 1978.
    _____

6   yours sincerely
    dr amy liu
    _____
    _____

7   she is from lismore which is in county waterford in ireland.
    _____

8 the faecal test returned a positive result for giardia intestinalis and i have organised repeat testing following treatment with flagyl, 400mg 3 times daily for 7 days.

9 ocean view respite care
15 kennedy terrace
beach bay
new south wales

10 the most recent outbreak of ebola began in the democratic republic of congo in august.

11 mr song is from south korea and requires an interpreter as he does not speak english.

12 we note from our records that you are now due for your routine dental examination.

WRITING PRACTICE 2: ERROR CORRECTION

Read the following sentences. Some are correct and some contain a word or words with incorrect capitalisation. If a sentence is correct, put a tick (✔) in the space provided at the end of the line. If a sentence is incorrect, rewrite the incorrect word or words using the correct capitalisation in the space provided at the end of the line. Two examples, (00) and (0), have been done for you.

00	Mrs Roxanne Ferguson is ready for transfer from Fairfield General Hospital to Cherry Park Aged Care Home.	✔
0	You are now due for your check-up at easy steps podiatry.	**Easy Steps Podiatry**
1	Mr Cranston's Blood Pressure has returned to normal.	
2	He was diagnosed with Huntington's Disease.	
3	The Physiotherapist recommended weight-bearing exercises to assist with Ms Brownlow's rehabilitation.	
4	Dr hill referred the patient to a dietician for advice on pre-operative weight loss.	
5	The nurse administered Ibuprofen for pain relief.	
6	Chickenpox is caused by the varicella-zoster virus.	
7	He was prescribed Phenergan for Allergic Rhinitis.	
8	Mr Martin was transported to hospital via Ambulance.	
9	His Spleen was removed laparoscopically.	
10	I am wondering if Ms Park is a suitable candidate for Laser Eye Surgery.	
11	Greenvale hospital has a specialist maternity ward.	
12	He will need to contact his personal doctor for the results of his tests.	

WRITING PRACTICE 3: USING CAPITAL LETTERS IN MEDICAL CORRESPONDENCE

Read Letter 1. This is a Letter of Referral from general practitioner Dr Alessio Greco to allergy specialist Dr Bruno Martini regarding patient Mr Dario Di Dio. The capital letters have been removed from the correspondence. Rewrite Letter 1 in the space provided to include capital letters where appropriate. The introduction to Letter 1 has been done for you as an example.

Letter 1: Read the Letter of Referral.

dr bruno martini

valley allergy specialists

suite 155, greenway house

56 market street

paddington

____ July 20___

dear bruno

re: dario di dio, aged 50

thank you for seeing mr dario di dio, aged 50 years, for allergy testing and management of his ongoing symptoms.

mr di dio has had intermittent nausea, headaches and fatigue for 2 years. the onset of symptoms occurred after an episode of gastroenteritis as a result of a helicobacter pylori infection.

i have performed a range of investigations, including a recent urea breath test to exclude h. pylori recurrence, the results of which were negative. copies are attached.

i have no other investigations planned at this time. as i have not found a clear pathology to target for treatment, i would be grateful for your specialist advice.

thank you for your care and management.

yours sincerely

dr alessio greco

Letter 1: Rewrite the Letter of Referral here using capital letters where appropriate.

Dr Bruno Martini

Valley Allergy Specialists

Suite 155, Greenway House

56 Market Street

Paddington

____ July 20____

Dear Bruno

Re: Mr Dario Di Dio, aged 50

Thank you for seeing Mr Dario Di Dio, aged 50 years, for allergy testing and management of his ongoing symptoms.

Read Letter 2. This is a clinical communication from allergy specialist Dr Bruno Martini to general practitioner Dr Alessio Greco regarding patient Mr Dario Di Dio. The capital letters have been removed from the correspondence. Rewrite Letter 2 in the space provided to include capital letters where appropriate.

Letter 2: Read the follow-up report.

Dr Alessio Greco

Family Medical Practice

97 Mulberry Terrace

Sunnyside

____ July 20___

Dear Alessio

Re: Mr Dario Di Dio

Dario Di Dio attended an appointment on May 19 to undergo allergy testing.

A skin prick test was used to test 32 potential allergens. Mr Di Dio tested positive to the dust mite allergen.

The recommended treatment is nasal rinsing with saline once per week using a commercially available product, an intranasal corticosteroid available over-the-counter, 2 sprays in each nostril, once per day, and dust mite protectors on all bedding including the mattress. (We recommend Allergex brand.)

If his symptoms fail to resolve, I recommend that Mr Di Dio should return to us for immunotherapy. This will involve one injection of a solution containing the dust mite allergen every month for 5 years.

I have also referred Mr Di Dio to dietician Giorgia Chiari for advice on commencing an elimination diet as his symptoms are also suggestive of a food chemical intolerance.

Thank you for referring this patient to Valley Allergy Specialists.

Yours sincerely

Dr Bruno Martini

Letter 2: Rewrite the follow-up report here using capital letters where appropriate.

UNIT 3 — DIABETES MANAGEMENT

STUDY FOCUS

Reading: Identifying main ideas and locating specific information
Vocabulary: Managing and exploring diabetes
Speaking: Identifying, acknowledging and incorporating the patient's perspective

Exploring the topic

In pairs or groups, discuss the following questions.

- What are the most common types of diabetes?
- How does diabetes affect the body?
- What treatments are available for diabetes?

STUDY BOOST 1: READING AND VOCABULARY

READING 1

Read Texts 1-6 and choose the most suitable answer A, B or C. An example (0) has been done for you.

BOOSTER TIP

For this task, identify **key words** in the questions and texts which will help you to locate the information you need to answer each question.

0 The diabetes information table indicates that the onset of type 2 diabetes usually occurs
   A   before the age of 40.
   B   at the age of 40.
   C   **after the age of 40.**

Diabetes information table		
	TYPE 1 - insulin dependent diabetes mellitus (IDDM)	TYPE 2 - non insulin dependent diabetes mellitus (NIDDM)
Age of onset	Usually <40	Usually >40
Onset	Sudden	Gradual
Insulin production	None or very little	Too little or ineffective
Symptoms	Blurry vision, frequent urination, increased appetite and thirst, mood changes and irritability, tiredness and weakness, unexplained weight loss	Increased appetite and thirst, dark patches on armpits and neck, frequent urination, blurry vision, tiredness and weakness, unexplained weight loss

Treatment	Healthy eating and meal planning, increased physical activity, blood glucose level checks, insulin injections or pump	Healthy eating and meal planning, increased physical activity, blood glucose level checks, oral medication may be needed, insulin injections may be needed

1   According to the pre-diabetes screening guide, one of the screening methods

    A   offers greater convenience for patients.

    B   is more accurate than the other tests.

    C   should always be repeated.

> **Pre-diabetes screening guide**
>
> To identify pre-diabetes, there are three blood testing methods which are currently recommended:
> - Fasting plasma glucose
> - 2-hour post 75g oral glucose challenge
> - HbA1c
>
> The HbA1c test does not require fasting or a lengthy stay at a pathology clinic and may be the preferred option for patients and physicians.
>
> It is important to note that for patients where the suspicion for pre-diabetes is high and test results return within the normal range, repeat testing within 12 months should be considered using one of the other two screening options.

2   According to the extract from the Clinical Practice Handbook, when a patient's blood glucose level (BGL) falls below 4mmol/L, the healthcare professional should

    A   administer fast-acting insulin.

    B   re-check the BGL after 15 grams of carbohydrate have been consumed.

    C   encourage the patient to drink diet soft drink.

> **Extract from Clinical Practice Handbook for Student Nurses:**
> **Nursing Interventions for type 1 diabetes patients**
>
> **HYPOGLYCAEMIA** occurs when a person's blood glucose level (BGL) has dropped below 4mmol/L. Hypoglycaemia must be treated quickly to prevent the BGL from falling further which may lead to loss of consciousness or seizures.
>
> If a patient's BGL has dropped below 4mmol/L, immediately give 15 grams of a fast-acting carbohydrate.
>
> Choose 1 of the following:
> - 6-7 jelly beans
> - 4-6 pieces of hard candy
> - 1/2 can of soft drink (NOT diet soft drink)
> - 1/2 glass fruit juice
> - 3 teaspoons of sugar or honey
> - glucose tablets or gel equivalent to 15 grams of carbohydrate

Check BGL again after 15 minutes.

If BGL remains at or below 4mmol/L, give another fast-acting carbohydrate and review BGL. If BGL has risen above 4mmol/L, provide one of the following as a snack:

- 1 slice of bread
- 1 glass of milk
- 1 piece of fruit
- dry biscuits
- 1 small tub of low-fat yoghurt

Ensure carbohydrate is included at the next meal. Pasta and rice are good options.

3 The guidelines for discharge planning require the healthcare professional to

    A   make arrangements for the patient to visit a diabetes care provider.

    B   confirm the patient is able to manage their illness.

    C   inform the patient of the costs of their hospital stay.

1 Guidelines for discharge planning for newly-diagnosed insulin-treated patients

1.3 Inpatient diabetes self-management education

- Assess the patient's level of understanding of their diabetes diagnosis
- Check the patient's understanding of self-monitoring of blood glucose, including indication, frequency, sites for testing and home blood glucose goals
- Determine the ability of the patient to conduct self-monitoring of blood glucose levels - supervise patient checking own blood glucose level
- Check knowledge of hyperglycaemia/hypoglycaemia - teach signs, symptoms, treatment and prevention
- Teach the patient when and how to administer medications, including method of administration and the proper use and disposal of needles and syringes
- Outline nutritional care plan, highlighting the importance of consistent eating patterns and carbohydrate counting
- Instruct the patient on the safe management of diabetes during periods of illness, specifically insulin dose adjustment and monitoring
- Provide contact details for a diabetes care provider

Note: Ongoing education and support will be provided by a dedicated diabetes health care team after discharge.

4 The excerpt from the Midwife Training Manual suggests that babies born to mothers with gestational diabetes may

   A   have diabetes at birth.
   B   be born with high blood glucose levels.
   C   suffer short-term adverse health effects.

Excerpt from Midwife Training Manual

Gestational Diabetes

There is a high risk of pre-term birth for women with gestational diabetes, although many pregnant women continue their pregnancy to full term and begin labour spontaneously.

There are health implications for babies of mothers with gestational diabetes. The baby can grow very large, increasing the likelihood of a problematic delivery which may result in the need for intervention with forceps or a vacuum device. For this reason, obstetricians may elect to deliver slightly before the due date by inducing labour or scheduling a caesarean section.

After the birth, there is a greater risk that these babies may develop jaundice and breathing difficulties, both of which are usually temporary, and may also struggle to feed. They may also have low blood glucose levels as they produce more insulin than is usual for a newborn baby. This is to compensate for the higher blood glucose levels in their mother's bloodstream.

Babies who require special care may be transferred to a neonatal intensive care unit (NICU) to ensure any problems that occur can be treated quickly. The baby will not be born with diabetes.

Blood glucose levels in the mother will usually return to normal after giving birth and most women will no longer have diabetes after the baby is born. There remains an increased possibility of gestational diabetes in subsequent pregnancies with both mother and baby having a greater risk of developing type 2 diabetes later in life.

5 The purpose of this email is to

   A   remind staff about procedures relating to blood glucose monitoring.
   B   highlight the need to involve residents in designing their care plans.
   C   schedule a medication review for residents with diabetes.

Blue Sky Care Home

Email

TO: All staff

SUBJECT: Blood glucose levels

A blood glucose monitoring routine is devised for each resident in consultation with the resident, their family and physician. Blood glucose monitoring routines are based on the individual needs of the resident and consider their personal circumstances.

All blood glucose measurements must be recorded in the appropriate chart. The resident's target range must be clearly written at the top of the chart and referred to at each measurement in line with their blood glucose management plan.

Any changes to the insulin regimen instigated by the resident or recommended by medical staff are to be documented in the chart and reported to the resident's physician for review.

6 The extract from Essential Medicine indicates that the first blood test in suspected cases of diabetic ketoacidosis (DKA) measures levels of

   A venous blood glucose.
   B arterial blood glucose.
   C capillary blood glucose.

> **Extract from Essential Medicine: Diabetes Mellitus**
>
> 6 Acute management of diabetic ketoacidosis (DKA) in adults
>
> 6.1 Diabetic ketoacidosis is a life-threatening emergency associated with significant mortality. Rapid assessment is essential as people with DKA can deteriorate very quickly.
>
> Initial point-of-care investigations to be undertaken:
> - A capillary (finger prick) blood glucose measurement (critical level >15mmol/L) should be taken. Ensure there is no sugar on the skin where the skin prick is made.
> - Capillary blood ketones (critical level >1.5mmol/L) should also be taken.
>
> Always follow this test with a formal venous blood glucose level test.
>
> Arterial blood is not needed as routine.
>
> In patients with elevated blood glucose levels and ketones who are not acidotic, close monitoring and aggressive management are essential to prevent progression to DKA.

VOCABULARY PRACTICE 1A: MATCHING MEANING

The words and phrases in Column A appear in Texts 1-6. Choose the most suitable word or phrase from Column B for each word or phrase in Column A. Write your answers in the space provided. An example (0) has been done for you.

COLUMN A		COLUMN B
0 **adjustment**	A	a procedure to test people for symptoms of a disease
1 subsequent	B	unclear, indistinct
2 consistent	C	can be potentially fatal, can result in death
3 compensate	D	actions taken to intercede to improve outcomes
4 aggressive	E	to reestablish a balance
5 interventions	F	**a minor modification**
6 life-threatening	G	constantly done in the same way
7 screening	H	a state of being unresponsive
8 instigated	I	initiated
9 loss of consciousness	J	intensive
10 blurry	K	following, occurring later

Write your answers here.

0	1	2	3	4	5	6	7	8	9	10
F										

VOCABULARY PRACTICE 1B: COMPLETE THE SENTENCE

For Questions 1-5, choose the most suitable word from the box to complete each sentence. There is one extra word that you do not need to use. An example (0) has been done for you.

> ~~consistent~~   screening   subsequent   instigated
> blurry   life-threatening   compensate

0   The patient's symptoms were **consistent** with a diagnosis of diabetes.

1   _____ to chemotherapy, the tumour had reduced to 60% of its original size.

2   Patients presenting with symptoms of fever, cough, sore throat, breathing difficulties are being referred to the dedicated COVID-19 _____ clinic.

3   Scientists have discovered that an improved sense of hearing may _____ for loss of sight.

4   The ophthalmologist advised the patient he would experience _____ vision after having drops instilled and should not drive for 4 hours.

5   If left untreated, chronic health conditions such as diabetes, asthma and cardiac disease may be _____.

READING 2

Read the text about living with type 1 diabetes. For Questions 1-5, choose the most suitable answer A, B or C. An example (0) has been done for you.

> **BOOSTER TIP**
>
> For this task, read the text carefully to locate the **specific information** required for each question. Read the details closely to ensure clear understanding of the text and questions.

Living with type 1 diabetes

'I was diagnosed with type 1 diabetes at the age of 11,' says Dr Linda Miller, a chemical pathologist, now aged 65. 'Treatment was basic back in those days and primarily involved using a special kind of test tape to check if glucose was present in urine, injecting fixed doses of insulin and frequently seeing the doctor.'

The way in which type 1 diabetes is managed has changed considerably since Dr Miller was diagnosed in 1957. Nowadays, precise doses of insulin can be calculated according to accurate blood glucose level readings and users have the choice of administering via a needle and syringe, an insulin pen or an insulin pump.

Significant technological advancements over the years, such as the development of continuous glucose monitoring (CGM) devices, have allowed diabetes patients greater independence to self-manage their disease. These CGM devices measure interstitial glucose levels in subcutaneous tissue rather than glucose levels in the blood. A tiny sensor attached to a transmitter is implanted under the skin to record glucose readings which are sent to a receiver for interpretation. If glucose levels drop or rise rapidly, CGM devices can trigger an alarm which alerts the patients to act quickly to prevent a hyperglycaemic or hypoglycaemic episode.

According to Dr Miller, incorporating continuous glucose monitoring into the diabetes care plan of young adults who require assistance with tracking their blood glucose levels improves glycaemic control.

A limitation of most CGM devices, however, is that they do not completely remove the need for capillary (finger prick) blood glucose testing using a blood glucose meter. This is because blood glucose meters provide more accurate results than continuous glucose monitoring, and are vital in situations where the glucose level is changing rapidly. Capillary blood glucose levels are also required to calibrate the CGM device at intervals determined by the manufacturer.

Flash glucose monitoring, which operates in much the same way as continuous glucose monitoring, involves a sensor being scanned with a reader or smart device to obtain a glucose level reading. Flash glucose monitoring (Flash GM) devices do not automatically alert the user if glucose levels are outside of the desired range. However, some brands of Flash GM devices allow users to program their device to activate an alarm if glucose levels become unstable.

In both CGM and Flash GM devices, blood glucose data can be sent to a smartphone app or other compatible device, allowing trends and patterns to be identified and giving users and their medical team valuable insight into how to best tailor treatment.

'A life-changing device for me personally has been a new type of insulin pump. One of the challenges of diabetes is delivering the correct dose of insulin at the time it is needed,' explains Dr Miller, who was fortunate to be one of the first patients to be fitted with the device.

The pump Dr Miller is referring to is a hybrid closed loop insulin pump system, which improves glycaemic control by continuously monitoring blood glucose levels and automatically adjusting the doses of insulin based on the readings. The insulin is then delivered into the body when it is required.

'Think of it as an artificial pancreas,' says Dr Miller. 'This technology will hopefully lead to fewer potentially dangerous fluctuations because blood glucose levels will be more stable.'

However, it is not yet a fully automatic system. The amount of carbohydrate consumed at mealtimes must be manually entered to calculate bolus insulin doses, which help to prevent blood glucose levels from becoming unstable. From a maintenance point of view, the sensor requires periodic calibration and parts may need to be repaired or replaced from time to time.

As for the future, Dr Miller remains optimistic. A new class of drug, baricitinib, currently used to treat rheumatoid arthritis, is being investigated for possible use by people with type 1 diabetes to protect insulin-producing cells from immune attack. It is hoped that, if successful, this drug will halt the progression of disease in people newly-diagnosed with diabetes.

'It's not a cure, but it's certainly a very promising step in that direction,' concludes Dr Miller.

Questions 1-5

0 When Dr Miller was first diagnosed with type 1 diabetes, the management of diabetes included

    A administering customised doses of insulin.

    B occasional consultations with the doctor.

    C regular testing for glucose in urine.

1 Dr Miller was born in

    A 1963.

    B 1946.

    C 1957.

2 Dr Miller supports including continuous glucose monitoring (CGM) in the diabetes care plan because
   A it enables patients to have more control over managing their condition.
   B patients no longer need to use capillary blood glucose testing.
   C young adult diabetes patients will avoid rapid changes in glucose levels.

3 Flash glucose monitoring (Flash GM) devices
   A send an instant warning to patients about changes in their glucose levels.
   B continuously display a patient's glucose level readings without scanning to a smart device.
   C provide useful data so doctors can offer the patient appropriate individualised treatment.

4 Dr Miller says the greatest benefit of the new hybrid insulin pump is that it
   A removes the need for the patient to manually calculate carbohydrate amounts consumed at mealtimes.
   B calculates and administers accurate doses of insulin into the body as and when required.
   C does not require any maintenance after being fitted to the patient.

5 Current research hopes to prove baricitinib that is effective in
   A preventing insulin-producing cells from being destroyed.
   B treating rheumatoid arthritis.
   C diagnosing people with type 1 diabetes.

VOCABULARY PRACTICE 2: WORD FORMS

For Questions 1-5, choose the most suitable answer A, B, or C to complete each sentence. An example (0) has been done for you.

0 X-ray images are sent to a radiographer for _____.
   A interpret   **B interpretation**   C interpreted

1 Medical device manufacturers recommend that devices should be professionally _____ at regular intervals to ensure accuracy.
   A calibrate   B calibration   C calibrated

2 After losing a tooth in an accident, the patient consulted a periodontist to discuss a dental _____.
   A implant   B implanting   C implanted

3 _____ advancements have had a significant impact on the lives of people with diabetes.
   A Technologically   B Technology   C Technological

4 _____ oestrogen levels may cause multiple symptoms in menopausal women.
   A Fluctuate   B Fluctuating   C Fluctuation

5 Living with a chronic illness can provoke a wide range of emotions, including anxiety, fear and _____.
   A depression   B depressing   C depressed

READING 3

Read the text about the prevention of diabetes complications. For Questions 1-10, choose the most suitable phrase (A-K) to complete each sentence. Write your answers in the space provided. An example (0) has been done for you.

The prevention of complications of diabetes

Chronic complications of type 1 diabetes are largely associated with **(0) <u>inadequate control of blood glucose levels (BGLs).</u>** BGLs which exceed the normal range over long periods of time can cause serious damage to large blood vessels (macrovascular), resulting in heart attack and stroke, and damage to (1) _____ (microvascular), which can lead to feet, eye and dental problems.

Patients who manage their diabetes well can significantly reduce the risk of serious complications, including (2) _____. Feet are particularly susceptible to diabetic nerve damage and (3) _____ to the feet and toes. For people with diabetes, this means they may not notice a cut or other minor injury to their feet, which should (4) _____. If these minor injuries do not heal, they can lead to serious infections, for example, ulcers (5) _____, which may result in amputation of toes, feet and other infected areas.

Recommended **foot care guidelines** for diabetes patients:

- Wash and clean feet every day and look for bruises, blisters or cuts.
- Cut toenails regularly.
- Ask a friend or family member to help you to (6) _____ and cut your toenails for you if you cannot see or touch your feet by yourself.
- Wear shoes and socks which maintain effective blood circulation and prevent damage to the feet.
- Visit a podiatrist to have your foot health assessed every six months.

Like diabetic neuropathy, diabetic retinopathy is also the result of raised BGLs over a long period, causing small blood vessels to the eye to weaken or become blocked. Treatment is required to prevent blurred vision or loss of vision. People with diabetes have an increased risk of developing cataracts. These may need to be surgically removed and (7) _____.

Recommended **eye care** guidelines for diabetes patients:

- Have regular eye checks every two years with an optometrist who will (8) _____.
- Visit an ophthalmologist for further specialist eye treatment if referred by the optometrist.

Patients with diabetes are strongly encouraged to be proactive in maintaining good dental health. If BGLs are not controlled, the high levels of glucose in the saliva will exacerbate the growth of bacteria in the mouth, causing mouth and gum infections, (9) _____ and 'oral burning'. Some initial symptoms of mouth problems include painful, swollen or bleeding gums.

Recommended **dental care** guidelines for diabetes patients:

- Brush teeth and floss daily.
- Drink water to stay hydrated and avoid sugary drinks.
- Visit a dentist for a complete mouth, (10) _____ with a professional clean every 6 months.

A assess any changes in your eye health
B and gangrene
C gum and teeth check-up
D replaced with an artificial intraocular lens (IOL)
E <u>inadequate control of blood glucose levels (BGLs)</u>
F such as gingivitis, periodontitis and xerostomia
G small blood vessels
H perform regular foot checks
I be treated
J diabetic neuropathy
K reduction in blood flow and sensation

Write your answers here.

0	1	2	3	4	5	6	7	8	9	10
E										

VOCABULARY PRACTICE 3: WORD FORMATION

Read the text about diabetic nephropathy. For Questions 1-10, write the correct form of the word given in bold to complete each sentence. You may need to check the words in a dictionary if you are unsure of the appropriate verb, noun, adjective or adverb form to use. An example (0) has been done for you.

DIABETIC NEPHROPATHY	
What is diabetic nephropathy?	
Diabetic nephropathy describes the chronic (0) <u>complication</u> of diabetes which damages the capillaries inside the kidneys after a (1) _____ period of elevated blood glucose levels (BGLs).	(0) complicate (1) prolong
What are common symptoms?	
Common symptoms of diabetic nephropathy include: • (2) _____ of the face, hands, ankles and feet from fluid (3) _____ • urinating more (4) _____ than normal • feeling tired and (5) _____	(2) swell (3) retain (4) frequent (5) nausea
How does it affect the body?	
Kidneys function as a (6) _____ system to excrete waste products and excess fluid from the body through urine.	(6) filter
Damage to the kidneys is (7) _____ through the amount of albumin found in urine samples.	(7) assess
(8) _____ of kidney disease into kidney (9) _____ indicates future dialysis or kidney transplant for the diabetes patient.	(8) progress (9) fail
How can risk factors be avoided?	
• Control BGLs, blood pressure, cholesterol levels • Exercise regularly and maintain a healthy (10) _____.	(10) weigh

Discussion

1 What essential information should be given to newly-diagnosed type 1 diabetes patients?
2 How important is it for diabetes patients to maintain good general health?
3 What impact have developments in technology had on the lives of diabetes patients?

STUDY BOOST 2: SPEAKING

Identifying, acknowledging and incorporating the patient's perspective

1 Communication strategies to elicit and explore the patient's perspective

Throughout the consultation, there will be opportunities to explore the patient's perspective through eliciting their ideas, concerns and expectations.

BEGINNING THE CONSULTATION

At the start of the consultation, using open questions will enable the healthcare professional to capture and explore the patient's perspective.

Examples

How can I help you today?
What can I help you with today?
What can I do for you today?

DURING THE CONSULTATION

As the consultation progresses, it is important to gather information from the patient in order to gain insight into their health and current condition.

Examples

How are you feeling generally?
What seems to make your symptoms better/worse?
How are your symptoms affecting your daily life?
Which symptoms are worrying you the most?
Tell me more about your symptoms.

Asking specific questions will help to explore how the patient may respond to a particular course of action.

Examples

<u>How do you feel about</u> *checking your own blood glucose levels?*
<u>Have you considered</u> *having a community nurse visit once per week?*

CONCLUDING THE CONSULTATION

At the end of the consultation, it is important that the patient feels that their expectations have been met in terms of addressing their concerns. This may include checking that they have understood what was discussed.

Examples

Does that all make sense?
Shall I summarise what we have talked about today?
Is there something else I can help you with?
Do you have any other concerns?

2 Communication strategies to acknowledge the patient's cues

Responding to verbal cues

Patients share their thoughts and feelings directly through spoken language and indirectly through non-verbal facial expressions and gestures.

In terms of recognising spoken cues, it is important to indicate to the patient that you have heard what they have said and are incorporating their perspective into your responses. Repeating back key words or ideas that the patient has expressed will demonstrate that you have understood and are acknowledging what they have said.

Examples

Pet owner:	*I think the nurse had better hold my dog while he is being vaccinated.*
Veterinarian:	*Yes. I will ask the nurse to hold your dog for you.*
Patient:	*I am finding it really difficult to get out of a chair.*
Occupational therapist:	*Have you thought about a motorised armchair which will support you when you are trying to stand?*
Patient:	*I have been wondering if I should have a cholesterol check.*
Physician:	*Why are you specifically interested in a cholesterol check?*
Patient:	*I cannot do the squats you recommended.*
Physiotherapist:	*What are you finding difficult about the squats?*

Responding to non-verbal cues

Patients display non-verbal cues in a number of ways. Facial expressions and body language may reveal how a patient is feeling. Interpreting these non-verbal cues can help the healthcare professional to explore the patient's perspective more effectively.

Examples

You seem a little confused by the information I have given you.

I sense you have some concerns about what I have just told you.

I understand that this is frustrating.

You are very quiet. Is there anything else you would like to ask?

3 Communication strategies to relate explanations to identified patient needs

It is important for healthcare professionals to relate their explanations to the information gained from the patient. This helps the patient to understand the rationale for conclusions and decisions regarding their situation. It also reassures the patient that their perspective has been heard, understood and incorporated into the decision-making process.

Examples

<u>I understand (that)</u> *you have not had much time to do these exercises, so let us do them together now.*

<u>I know (that)</u> *you do not like needles, but an intravenous iron infusion will help you to feel so much better as you are anaemic.*

<u>You mentioned (that)</u> *you drink a lot of fruit juice. I need to tell you it is damaging the enamel on your teeth.*

<u>You said (that)</u> *you find it difficult to breathe when lying down. We need to investigate why.*

SPEAKING PRACTICE 1: CHOOSE THE APPROPRIATE RESPONSE

Match the sentences in Column A with the most suitable response in Column B. Write your answers in the space provided. An example (0) has been done for you.

COLUMN A PATIENT	COLUMN B HEALTHCARE PROFESSIONAL
0 **I am worried that the ECG will hurt.**	A What would you like to ask first?
1 I have not seen you for a while. I have a lot of questions for you.	B Yes, that is right. I will be back to shower you soon.
2 I thought I would be running again by now.	C Shaky? You had better sit down while I examine you.
3 I am wondering if there is another way to control the pain.	D **No, it is pain-free. It will not hurt at all.**
4 I am not sure if I understand.	E I will check your temperature in a moment.
5 The deep breathing exercises are really painful. I do not like doing them.	F Running? Well, we are working towards that.
6 I am feeling very shaky this morning.	G Unfortunately, it is not suitable for you, but there are other types of eye surgery which may help.
7 I thought you were giving me a shower this morning.	H Well, how do you feel about checking your own blood pressure at home?
8 I would like to ask about laser eye surgery.	I Would you like me to explain it again?
9 Do I need to come in every day to have my blood pressure checked?	J Another way? We can try a different medication.
10 I think I might have a fever.	K I understand the deep breathing exercises are painful, but, in your case, they are really important to help prevent pneumonia.

Write your answers here.

0	1	2	3	4	5	6	7	8	9	10
D										

SPEAKING PRACTICE 2: WHAT WOULD YOU SAY?

What would you say to show you are understanding and incorporating the patient's perspective in the following situations?

1. a patient who is expecting an expired prescription to be dispensed
2. a patient who does not appear to understand the explanation you have given
3. a patient who wants an immediate diagnosis but needs to undergo testing
4. a claustrophobic patient who is reluctant to have magnetic resonance imaging (MRI)
5. a patient with multiple symptoms who does not know what to discuss first
6. a patient who is deep in thought and quiet at the end of the consultation

SPEAKING PRACTICE 3: ROLE PLAY

ROLE PLAY 1

Work in pairs as healthcare professional and patient. Read your role play card to familiarise yourself with the task. Take a few minutes to plan what you are going to say. You can make notes during the preparation time if you wish.

> **BOOSTER TIP**
>
> For this task, demonstrate that you have identified, acknowledged and incorporated the patient's perspective into your responses.

ROLE PLAY 1

ROLE A: HEALTHCARE PROFESSIONAL SETTING: MATERNITY CLINIC

Your 30-year-old patient is at 26 weeks' gestation and has recently been diagnosed with gestational diabetes after failing a routine oral glucose tolerance test. The patient is feeling anxious about the diagnosis. You are going to speak to the patient about managing the condition.

TASK

- Find out what the patient knows about her gestational diabetes diagnosis.
- Ask about symptoms.
- Advise the patient that she should not require insulin. The condition will be managed by following a low GI diet.
- Inform the patient that she will need to test her blood glucose levels 4 times per day. Explain how to measure blood glucose levels, including the need to do a fasting test first thing in the morning. The remaining tests should be taken 2 hours after meals.
- Inform the patient what their target blood glucose range is. The fasting level must be less than 5.0mmol/L. The post-meal level must be less than 6.7mmol/L.
- Advise the patient what they should do if they have an elevated blood glucose level reading. (Keep a written record of blood glucose level readings and contact your diabetes educator if you have two high readings in a 7-day period.)
- Tell the patient to contact the maternity clinic at any time if they have concerns.
- Reassure the patient that the condition usually resolves following childbirth. A repeat oral glucose tolerance test will be conducted 6 weeks after delivery to check that the condition has resolved.

ROLE PLAY 1

ROLE B: PATIENT SETTING: MATERNITY CLINIC

You are 30 years old and 26 weeks pregnant. You have recently been diagnosed with gestational diabetes. You have not noticed any symptoms. You are feeling anxious about the diagnosis. A healthcare professional is going to speak to you about managing your condition.

TASK

- When asked, say that you know that you have gestational diabetes and you know little about the condition.
- If asked about your symptoms, explain that you have not noticed any symptoms.
- Appear concerned that your condition will be managed through diet alone as you believed diabetes should always be treated with insulin.
- Act surprised when told you need to check your blood glucose levels 4 times per day.
- Appear overwhelmed by the amount of information you are given regarding checking your blood glucose levels.
- Tell the healthcare professional that you do not feel confident about self-monitoring your condition.
- Ask if you will have gestational diabetes after you give birth.

ROLE PLAY 2

Work in pairs as healthcare professional and patient. Read your role play card to familiarise yourself with the task. Take a few minutes to plan what you are going to say. You can make notes during the preparation time if you wish.

ROLE PLAY 2

ROLE A: HEALTHCARE PROFESSIONAL **SETTING: MEDICAL CLINIC**

Your patient is 22 years old, morbidly obese and was diagnosed with type 2 diabetes 3 years ago. He/She has been advised in previous consultations to make significant lifestyle modifications to avoid medication and potential diabetes-related complications in the future.

TASK

- Ask whether your patient has adopted any of the recommended lifestyle changes.
- Ask your patient what changes he/she has made to his/her diet.
- Remind your patient that he/she needs to decrease fat intake, increase fibre intake, eat smaller portions and consume fewer calories.
- Ask your patient how much exercise he/she does in a week.
- Remind your patient that he/she should aim for a minimum of 30 minutes of moderate intensity physical activity per day and a 30-minute session of high intensity exercise per week.
- Ask your patient if he/she has managed to stop smoking.
- Recommend a program to stop smoking.
- Ask how much sleep your patient has. The goal is 6-9 hours per night.
- Find out how your patient manages stress. Stress management is important for people with diabetes. Your patient should consider using mindfulness techniques to manage stress.
- Suggest counselling with a specialist diabetes educator to help your patient to develop a plan to implement the recommended lifestyle changes.

ROLE PLAY 2

ROLE B: PATIENT **SETTING: MEDICAL CLINIC**

You are 22 years old and have had type 2 diabetes for 3 years. You enjoy going to parties with friends, socialising and staying up late. At previous appointments, you have been instructed to change your lifestyle to include eating healthier food, taking regular exercise and stopping smoking. However, you have not made any changes.

TASK

- Be defensive when explaining that you have not made any of the recommended changes to your lifestyle. You feel that your type 2 diabetes diagnosis is not affecting your health.

- When asked, say that you have not made any changes to your diet. You live with friends and you all eat a lot of fast food and high calorie snacks. It is too time-consuming to make home-cooked meals for yourself.

- Agree to make some changes to your diet.

- When asked, say that you do no regular exercise, but you dance at parties.

- When asked, say that you only smoke occasionally.

- When asked, say you usually sleep for about 9 hours per night.

- When asked, say you manage stress by spending time with friends and relaxing.

- When advised to undergo counselling, question the need for counselling and say that you do not think it is necessary at this stage.

UNIT 4 | FOCUS ON COMMON ERRORS 1: SPELLING

STUDY FOCUS

Writing: Developing awareness of using accurate and standardised spelling in medical documentation to achieve clear communication.

Recognising and avoiding spelling errors in frequently-occurring words.

Exploring the topic

In pairs or groups, discuss the following questions.

- What medical documents are you required to write as part of your healthcare role?
- What do you do to check that the spelling in the documents you write is accurate?
- What are some words that you often spell incorrectly?

STUDY BOOST 1

Recognising spelling errors in medical terms that can cause confusion

Information recorded in medical documentation must provide a clear and accurate account of a patient's history.

The accurate spelling of the language used in medical documents is essential to support clarity of communication. Although some medical terms have a similar spelling, they refer to completely different diseases, medications, parts of the body or treatments. For example: anuresis describes being unable to urinate and enuresis refers to passing urine while sleeping (wetting the bed).

Using a misspelled medical term could cause confusion and lead to critical miscommunication between healthcare professionals or between healthcare professionals and patients.

Task 1

Look at the pairs of medical terms (1-10) in Column A in the table. Choose the most suitable description from Column B for each word in Column A. Write your answers in the space provided. Two examples (00) and (0) have been done for you.

BOOSTER TIP
If you are unsure of the correct spelling of the medical term you want to use, it is essential to check the word in a medical reference text or dictionary.

COLUMN A		COLUMN B
00 **deceased**	A	a part of the male reproductive system
0 **diseased**	B	a non-cancerous fatty lump of tissue under the skin
1 palpation	C	a condition where inflamed arteries cause decreased blood flow to organs
2 palpitation	D	a cancer which originates in lymph glands
3 ileum	E	lying in a face-down position
4 ilium	F	a rapid, irregular heartbeat caused by anxiety, illness or exercise
5 arteritis	G	**no longer living**
6 arthritis	H	the largest part of hip bone
7 prostrate	I	the longest section of small intestine
8 prostate	J	a condition causing swelling, pain and stiffness in joints
9 lipoma	K	**suffering from/affected by an illness, ailment**
10 lymphoma	L	using hands to identify an organ or locate the source of pain in physical examinations

Write your answers here.

00	0	1	2	3	4	5	6	7	8	9	10
G	K										

STUDY BOOST 2

Avoiding spelling errors in frequently-occurring words

While there are many spelling rules available to help you to avoid making spelling errors, there are some words in English that do not follow standard spelling patterns and can cause difficulty for learners.

In your writing, you may choose to use standardised British spelling conventions or American spelling conventions. The most important point to remember is to use one style consistently. Do not confuse the two styles.

Task 2

Look carefully at the table with examples of frequently-used words and the patterns of spelling changes required when using different forms of these words. Highlight the words that you might find useful to focus on in your own writing.

BOOSTER TIP

When you meet a new word:

- look up the base word in a dictionary.
- note the spelling changes of the base word when transformed into other common forms, for example, an adjective, noun, verb or adverb.
- record the word in your 'Personal common error register' (see template in Answer Key).
- practise using the new word in your own writing.

Table: Examples of common words with some spelling pattern changes for different forms

Base words	Making changes to base word forms *Note: spelling changes*	Base words	Making changes to base word forms *Note: spelling changes*
'r' or 'rr'		**Plural nouns with 'ty' and 'py' ending**	
refer/reference	referring/referral/	disability	disabilities
occur	occurrence	therapy	therapies
Change final 't' to 'ce'		**-ibe to -iption**	
absent	absence	prescribe	prescription
present	presence	subscribe	subscription
-ance suffixes		**-ence suffixes**	
assist	assistance	independent	independence
attend	attendance	negligent	negligence
ate to -ation		**More changes before adding -ation**	
resuscitate	resuscitation	administer	administration
medicate	medication	calcify	calcification
vaccinate	vaccination	inflame	inflammation

-ic at end of word		-le to -ility	
trauma	traumatic	mobile	mobility
strategy	strategic	sterile	sterility
haemorrhage	haemorrhagic	vulnerable	vulnerability
British spelling		**American spelling**	
(-ise)		(-ize)	
mobilise	mobilisation	mobilize	mobilization
hospitalise	hospitalisation	hospitalize	hospitalization
sanitise	sanitisation	sanitize	sanitization
(-ce/se)		(-ce)	
practice (noun)	practise (verb)	practice (noun and verb)	
licence (noun)	license (verb)	licence (noun and verb)	

WRITING PRACTICE 1: SPOT THE ERROR

Look at the words in the box below. Decide which words are correctly spelled, and which words contain spelling errors. Copy the correctly spelled words from the box into Column A in the table. Underline the words in the box that contain mistakes and write the correct spelling of these words in Column B in the table. Two examples (00) and (0) have been done for you.

reference   reccommendation   attendance   **importence**   prescribe
inhibitor   specialize   strategy   **beginning**   artificil
ajustment   subscription   asociation   maintenance   vacinate
resussitate   accomodation   stability   mobilise   refering
inflamation   sustenance   occurrence   negligent   unecessary

Write your answers here.

COLUMN A: WORDS SPELLED CORRECTLY IN BOX ✔	COLUMN B: REWRITE INCORRECTLY SPELLED WORDS IN BOX USING CORRECT SPELLING.
(00) beginning	(0) importance

WRITING PRACTICE 2: ERROR CORRECTION

Read the following correspondence between Dr Atkinson and Dr Fulcher (Letter 1 and Letter 2) regarding Mrs Florence Hopkins.

Mrs Florence Hopkins is the patient. Dr Fulcher is the referring dentist. Dr Atkinson is the endodontist.

Look at the spelling of each word in each line of Letter 1 and Letter 2. Some lines are correct. Some lines contain words which are spelled incorrectly. If a line is correct, put a tick (✓) in the space provided at the end of the line. If a line contains a word that is spelled incorrectly, write the correct spelling of that word at the end of the line. An example (0) has been done for you.

Letter 1 - Letter of Referral from dentist to endodontist

	Dear Dr Atkinson Re: Mrs Florence Hopkins (DOB: 05/05/1955)	
0	Thank you for seeing Mrs Hopkins who preesented to my clinic today	**presented**
1	with a suspected fracture to tooth 17. Mrs Hopkins is expercing pain and	
2	sensitivity in the region of tooth 17 and as such was unwilling to allow me	
3	to examine the tooth. I have discussed the managment of tooth 17 with Mrs	
4	Hopkins, including the liklihood of the need for extraction. However, Mrs	
5	Hopkins is reluctant and would like to preserve the integrety of the tooth	
6	if possible. Mrs Hopkins is taking paracetamol (Calpol) 500mg x2 as needed	
7	(maximum 8 tablets per day), to manage the pain. I have prescribed	
8	amoxicillin, (Amoxil) 250mg every 8 hours, to prevent infecion.	
9	I would be grateful if you could provide further assesment of Mrs Hopkins	
10	and discuss treatment options with her in relation to potentially saving this	
11	tooth. Please do not hesetate to contact me if you require any information.	
12	Yours sincerly Dr Fulcher	

Letter 2 - Letter from endodontist to dentist

	Dear Dr Fulcher **Re: Mrs Florence Hopkins (DOB: 05/05/1955)**
13	Thank you for refering Mrs Hopkins in relation to the appropriate treatment
14	of tooth 17. On examination, tooth 17 has a fracture below the gum line,
15	hence, the seviere sensitivity she is experiencing. Due to extensive damage
16	to the structure of the tooth, I have adviced Mrs Hopkins that the tooth
17	should be extracted at her earliest convenience. I have instructed Mrs
18	Hopkins to continue with the antibiotics as a precautionery measure.
19	Analgesia may be taken as required. Mrs Hopkins will follow up with you
20	to arange the extraction of this tooth.
21	Yours sinceeley Dr Atkinson

UNIT 5 — CONSOLIDATION 1 (UNITS 1-4)

READING PRACTICE

Texts A-D relate to arthritis conditions. Read Texts A-D and answer Questions 1-20.

TEXT A: Rheumatoid Arthritis

Although rheumatoid arthritis cannot be cured, treatments are available which will reduce pain and swelling in the affected joints. With effective treatment, the disease can be kept in remission for periods of time. Flare-ups of intense pain and reduced mobility in the joints, however, may still occur from time-to-time, causing patients to experience difficulty with daily tasks, such as showering and dressing. During episodes of active rheumatoid arthritis, sufferers may experience more pronounced morning joint stiffness.

An early start to the treatment of rheumatoid arthritis following diagnosis is understood to reduce the risk of severe joint damage and disability. Initial treatment typically includes methotrexate or another DMARD (disease-modifying antirheumatic drug), which acts to suppress the body's immune and inflammatory responses. However, as this medication takes 3-6 weeks before any effect on symptom relief is noticed, a corticosteroid may be temporarily prescribed.

Research continues to explore a potential link between diet and triggers of arthritis pain and inflammation. Dieticians recommend that rheumatoid arthritis patients follow a diet of fresh fruit and vegetables, chicken and foods rich in omega-3 fatty acids, while avoiding typical triggers of arthritis inflammation, such as processed or sugary foods, red meat and alcohol. They further suggest that patients might find it helpful to complete an elimination diet to discover which foods stimulate an inflammatory response.

Regular low-impact exercise, such as yoga, swimming and walking in addition to maintaining a healthy weight and cardiovascular health are equally strongly advised as there is an increased risk of heart disease linked to rheumatoid arthritis.

TEXT B: Osteoarthritis

- long-term condition - commonly affects older adults
- generally affects joints including knees, hips and hands
- does not usually affect shoulders, elbows or wrists
- also known as 'wear and tear' arthritis - caused by gradual deterioration of cartilage in joints which protects ends of bones from scraping against each other
- sometimes produces a grating or cracking sound, known as crepitus, when patients mobilise arthritic joints

Common symptoms

- pain, swelling, redness, reduced flexibility in joints
- morning pain with joint stiffness - generally eases about 30 minutes after patient becomes active
- sleep interrupted by pain for sufferers with advanced osteoarthritis

Treatments available

- non-steroidal anti-inflammatory drugs (NSAIDs) to manage pain and reduce inflammatory heat and swelling in joints
- specific physiotherapy to assist with pain management
- cortisone injections into joint (maximum 3-4 per year) to reduce pain for a few weeks
- surgery – including total knee or hip replacement - to relieve long-term inflammation and pain and restore flexibility of movement

TEXT C: Polymyalgia Rheumatica (PMR)

1. Patient: Mrs Ethel Stolly (70 years)

2. On presentation:
- sudden onset of intense pain in shoulders
- significant reduction of flexibility in shoulder muscles, neck and hips on both sides of body
- highest pain level and muscle stiffness in mornings for about 45 minutes
- unable to dress and shower without assistance
- extreme tiredness

3. Blood tests:

Tests	Results	Range
Erythrocyte sediment rate (ESR)	8mm/hr	(1-29)
C-reactive protein (CRP)	+19mg/L	(0-6)

4. Diagnosis: Following physical examination of the symptoms and the elevated level of inflammation shown in the CRP test results, a diagnosis of polymyalgia rheumatica (PMR) was confirmed.

5. Treatment: Steroid medication (prednisolone) prescribed to reduce inflammation - initial dose 40mg per day taken with food for 5 days. Gradually reduced to reach a short-term maintenance dose of between 5-20mg per day to suppress the return of PMR symptoms. For long-term use, alternate day therapy is preferred.

6. Prognosis: very good with early diagnosis and appropriate therapy. Patient may require ongoing treatment 2-3 years until the disease recedes completely. Treatment should not be stopped suddenly or without medical advice. Flare-ups of PMR may occur if the medication is reduced too quickly. Ongoing medical supervision of patient with regular assessment of treatment and blood tests to investigate inflammation levels is essential. Patient advised to seek urgent medical advice if experiencing severe headache, which does not respond to pain relief, or notices any change to vision.

TEXT D: Juvenile Arthritis (JA) – paediatric rheumatic disease

Children and teenagers living with a chronic disease, such as juvenile arthritis, are very likely to suffer from anxiety and depression. Although individual reactions will vary, typical emotional and behavioural patterns are observed from initial diagnosis to understanding and acceptance.

1. Initial diagnosis of juvenile arthritis brings uncertainty, anxiety and fear. The young newly-diagnosed patient and the family may feel bewildered, as they try to process the information about the disease and understand the changes it will present.

    The diagnosis raises key questions for:

The patient	The family
• why me? • what can I do? • will the disease and the pain go away? • will my friends still want to socialise with me?	• how can they help the patient to adjust to living with the disease? • what is the most effective strategy to help the patient stay active, social and positive?

2. As the patient starts to realise the impact of the disease on everyday life, s/he may feel:
    - frustrated with the ongoing chronic pain and the reliance on pain relief medication.
    - angry that full participation in some favourite activities is no longer possible.
    - worried about being 'different' from peers.

3. If the juvenile patient becomes overwhelmed while trying to adapt to the changes associated with the disease, family members may observe:
    - isolation/withdrawal from family and friends.
    - behavioural differences, including mood swings.
    - poor appetite.
    - interrupted sleep patterns.
    - depression.

4. The juvenile patient needs assistance to move forward with a positive mindset.
    - Families can help the patient choose activities that can be managed within the limitations of the disease.
    - Support groups can encourage the patient to join social activities with other juvenile patients who also suffer from chronic pain conditions.
    - Psychotherapists can help with depression through mindfulness techniques, cognitive therapy to talk about thoughts and feelings related to the situation and behavioural therapy to discuss what changes are possible to make the situation more manageable.

Questions 1-8

Decide in which text A, B, C or D you can find the information mentioned in Questions 1- 8. You may refer to each text more than once. Write your answers in the space provided. An example (0) has been done for you.

In which text can you find information about:

0 particular foods which can aggravate arthritis inflammation and pain?
1   a treatment which should be decreased slowly under medical supervision?
2   a surgical procedure as a solution to improving joint mobility?
3   patients who stop socialising with friends?
4   a non-surgical treatment that has a recommended annual limit on the frequency of administration?
5   a range of counselling therapies?
6   keep-fit activities which are recommended?
7   a noise which may be heard in joints when a patient moves?
8   treatment that is recommended every second day?

Write your answers here.

0	1	2	3	4	5	6	7	8
A								

Questions 9-15

Answer Questions 9-15 with a word or short phrase from Texts A - D. Each answer may include words, numbers or both.

9   What symptoms experienced by a patient with a chronic arthritis condition require immediate medical attention?
_____

10 How long is a DMARD (disease-modifying antirheumatic drug) usually taken before evidence of improving symptoms is noticeable to patients?
_____

11 What is being checked in x-rays of the joints in the knee and the hip?
_____

12 What are two behaviours that indicate mental health challenges in young patients suffering from chronic pain?
_____ and _____

13 How can patients assess which foods contribute to their pain and inflammation?
_____

14 Which time of the day do arthritis patients most need assistance with their personal hygiene routines?
_____

15 What does a C-reactive protein (CRP) test result of 19mg/L in a patient presenting with arthritis symptoms indicate?
_____

Questions 16-20

Complete Questions 16-20 by using a word or short phrase from Texts A-D. Each answer may include words, numbers or both.

16 Psychotherapists encourage young patients suffering from chronic pain to think positively about new ways _____ their situation more easily.

17 As arthritis patients have a greater _____ disease, they are advised to eat healthy foods, exercise regularly and maintain quality sleep patterns.

18 Non-steroidal anti-inflammatory drugs (NSAIDs) can help with pain management and reduction of _____ and swelling in joints.

19 A key objective of early diagnosis and prompt commencement of effective treatment for arthritis sufferers is to _____ to the joint.

20 The recommended short-term maintenance treatment to prevent symptoms of a PMR relapse is _____ mg steroid medication (e.g. prednisolone) per day.

WRITING PRACTICE 1: ERROR CORRECTION (CAPITAL LETTERS)

Read the following sentences in Letter 1. Some sentences are correct and some contain one word with incorrect capitalisation. If a sentence is correct, put a tick (✔) in the space provided at the end of the line. If a sentence is incorrect, rewrite the incorrect word using the correct capitalisation in the space provided at the end of the line. Two examples, (00) and (0), have been done for you.

Letter 1: Referral from general practitioner (GP) to physiotherapist

00	Dear dylan	Dylan
0	I am writing to introduce Ms Cressida Brown who requires support to manage the symptoms she is experiencing in relation to her left knee joint.	✔
1	Ms Brown has clinical signs of Osteoarthritis in her left knee, including crepitus and swelling around the joint.	
2	she complains of flexion pain, notably when ascending and descending stairs.	
3	She reports joint instability at times and I wonder if she also has a patella tracking disorder.	
4	I would be grateful for your assessment and advice on how to best manage Ms Brown's symptoms.	
5	I have discussed the benefits of Physiotherapist input with her.	
6	I have prescribed meloxicam, (moxicam) 15mg daily, as necessary, to relieve any pain.	
7	Thank you for seeing this patient.	
8	Please contact me should you require further information.	
9	Yours Sincerely	
10	dr Romala Pitu	

WRITING PRACTICE 2: ERROR CORRECTION (SPELLING)

Read the following sentences in Letter 2. Some sentences are correct and some contain one word with incorrect spelling. If a sentence is correct, put a tick (✔) in the space provided at the end of the line. If a sentence is incorrect, rewrite the incorrect word using the correct spelling in the space provided at the end of the line. Two examples, (00) and (0), have been done for you.

Letter 2: Letter from physiotherapist to general practitioner (GP)

00	Dear Dr Pitu	✔
0	Thank you for refering Ms Brown for review and treatment.	**referring**
1	On examination, there was tenderness and pain on joint line pallpation.	
2	Pain increased on passive extension.	
3	I suspect areas of cartiledge loss.	
4	There is evidence of soft tissue oedema.	
5	The medial and lateral menissci appear to be intact as are the ACL, MCL and LCL.	
6	There may be a low-grade partial thickness tear to the proximal PCL.	
7	This is unrelated to the osteoarthritis diagnosis and may have been susstained when twisting the knee during a recent game of netball.	
8	Further investigations including x-ray and MRI may be indicated.	
9	Ms Brown is unable to weigt bear on the affected leg and the joint is very unstable.	
10	With regards to the joint instability, I feel this is related to muscle weakness around the joint, rather than a seperate patella tracking problem.	
11	Ms Brown attended 3 sessions and her symptyms have somewhat reduced.	
12	I prescribed a home exercise program focussing on strengthening and balance exercises and reccomended icing the joint at night.	
13	I have concluded our sessions as Ms Brown has made good progress.	
14	Going forward, Ms Brown will do a weekly pilates class under the supervision of a physiotherapist.	
15	I have adviced Ms Brown that stationary cycling to increase quadricep muscle and tendon strength would also be beneficial.	
16	I have discussed with Ms Brown the importance of long-term complaince with an exercise program to optimise function and manage pain.	
17	If you require further infromation, please do not hesitate to contact me.	
18	Yours sinceerely Dylan Bradbury	

SPEAKING PRACTICE: INCORPORATING THE PATIENT'S PERSPECTIVE

ROLE PLAY 1

Work in pairs as healthcare professional and patient. Read your role play card to familiarise yourself with the task. Take a few minutes to plan what you are going to say. You can make notes during the preparation time if you wish.

ROLE PLAY 1

ROLE A: HEALTHCARE PROFESSIONAL   **SETTING: FAMILY HEALTH CARE CLINIC**

Your 25-year-old patient presents with fatigue. You suspect that the fatigue is related to the patient's lifestyle. You would like your patient to have a blood test in order to assess their general health. Your patient is nervous about having a blood test.

TASK

- Find out about your patient's symptoms.

- Explain that ongoing fatigue in a young adult is usually related to lifestyle factors. Offer advice on leading a healthy lifestyle (e.g. sleep, exercise, diet, work/life balance).

- Inform your patient that you would like to order a blood test as a first step to gain insight into his/her overall health and exclude physical causes of fatigue.

- Explain that fatigue as a symptom on its own is rarely due to an underlying illness.

- Acknowledge that your patient feels anxious about having a blood test and convince him/her that it needs to be done. Emphasise that a blood test is quite quick, minimally invasive and the staff are trained to minimise any discomfort.

- Reassure your patient that you will call him/her to discuss the results of the blood test and that you will investigate further after you have a clearer picture of their general health.

ROLE PLAY 1

ROLE B: PATIENT   **SETTING: FAMILY HEALTH CARE CLINIC**

You are 25 years old and have been feeling unusually tired for about 3 months. You otherwise feel well. The healthcare professional is requesting that you have a blood test. You are nervous about having a blood test and do not think it is necessary.

TASK

- When asked, say that you have felt more tired than usual for several months. You do not have any other symptoms.

- Become defensive when offered lifestyle advice. You feel that you lead a healthy lifestyle overall. Admit that you have been working long hours.

- When told that you need a blood test, say that you are worried that the healthcare professional suspects a serious health problem.

- Resist attempts to persuade you that you need a blood test.

- Reluctantly agree to have a blood test.

- Appear reassured that the healthcare professional will contact you with the results of the blood test.

ROLE PLAY 2

Work in pairs as healthcare professional and parent of patient. Read your role play card to familiarise yourself with the task. Take a few minutes to plan what you are going to say. You can make notes during the preparation time if you wish.

ROLE PLAY 2

ROLE A: HEALTHCARE PROFESSIONAL **SETTING: PAEDIATRIC WARD**

You are talking to the parent of a 7-year-old child with a persistent lower respiratory infection which is suggestive of atypical pneumonia. The child is scheduled to have a bronchoscopy to investigate the cause of the infection. You are answering the parent's questions prior to the procedure.

TASK

- Find out if the parent has any questions regarding the procedure.

- Explain why bronchoscopy is indicated – the child has a persistent infection that is not responding to antibiotics and bronchoscopy is the next step. Bronchoscopy provides clinically important information which will assist with diagnosis and treatment.

- Briefly explain that a sample of lung fluid (bronchoalveolar lavage) and a sample of lung tissue (biopsy) will be taken which will hopefully identify the cause of the infection.

- Reassure the parent that bronchoscopy is a safe, well-tolerated procedure.

- Inform the parent that their child will be sedated and they will not experience any discomfort.

- Inform the parent that significant haemorrhage following lung biopsy is rare; symptoms of haemoptysis (coughing up blood) typically resolve on their own without medical intervention.

- When asked, inform the parent that following the procedure the child will be transferred from theatre to a recovery room where they will be observed closely for 30 minutes. Oxygen levels will be monitored. The doctor who performed the procedure will speak to the parent afterwards.

- Resist the request to discharge the patient. (The child needs to remain in hospital while the pneumonia is being treated.)

ROLE PLAY 2

ROLE B: PARENT OF PATIENT **SETTING: PAEDIATRIC WARD**

You are the parent of a 7-year-old child who requires a bronchoscopy to investigate the cause of a persistent respiratory infection. You are talking to a healthcare professional about your concerns prior to the procedure.

TASK

- Ask if there is a less invasive way to investigate your child's illness.
- Ask what the procedure involves.
- Say that you are worried about the safety of the procedure.
- Say that you are concerned that the procedure will be painful.
- Admit that you are worried about internal bleeding following a biopsy.
- Ask what happens immediately after the procedure.
- Say that you would like to take your child home after the procedure.

UNIT 6 GASTROINTESTINAL INVESTIGATIONS

STUDY FOCUS

Reading: Identifying main ideas and locating specific information
Vocabulary: Investigating gastrointestinal symptoms
Writing: Organising a medical letter

Exploring the topic

In pairs or groups, discuss the following questions.

- What are some illnesses that affect the gastrointestinal tract?
- What symptoms are typically associated with gastrointestinal complaints?
- What investigations may be recommended for suspected gastrointestinal illnesses?

STUDY BOOST 1: READING AND VOCABULARY

READING 1

Task 1

Texts A-D relate to investigations into gastrointestinal symptoms. Choose the most suitable heading (i-iv) for each text from the list in the box and write the heading on the line provided.

BOOSTER TIP

For this task, read quickly to identify the **main idea** of the text. You do not need to focus on all of the information given.

HEADINGS

i) ULTRASOUND OF UPPER ABDOMEN
ii) CANINE INFECTIOUS AGENTS SCREENING
iii) FOOD CHEMICAL ELIMINATION PLAN
iv) PATHOLOGY TEST RESULTS

TEXT A: _____

Eat only foods from the strict and moderate categories of the baseline diet, including gluten-free foods, for the next 3 weeks. Commence the amine challenge after 21 days on the baseline diet.

Amine challenge - choose at least 2 serves per day from the list below:

- 1-2 bananas (any ripeness)
- good quality milk chocolate/cocoa in baking or hot chocolate drink
- nitrate-free ham/bacon
- tinned salmon/tuna in springwater, unflavoured
- 120g of any cut of pork or roast chicken (with skin)
- tasty cheddar cheese

Continue the amine challenge for 7 days. Make note of any reaction (headaches, fatigue, nausea, diarrhoea) you have during the challenge. Cease the challenge if symptoms become severe. At the end of the amine challenge, return to the baseline diet for 3 days unless a reaction occurs. It is ideal to experience 3 consecutive days without symptoms before proceeding with the salicylate challenge.

TEXT B: _____

Name of Test: MULTIPLEX VET FAECAL PCR

Salmonella spp. DNA	Not Detected
Campylobacter jejuni DNA	Not Detected
Cryptosporidium canis DNA	Not Detected
Giardia spp. DNA	Not Detected
Parvovirus DNA	Not Detected
Coronavirus RNA	Detected

This test is designed to screen for a panel of multiple infectious agents through a single faecal sample.

Although the reagents are designed using consensus nucleic acid sequences and validated to detect all of the infectious agents mentioned above, it is worthwhile noting that there may be some genetic variants which may escape detection by this methodology.

A PCR positive result should be interpreted with reference to other clinical data, including clinical signs and vaccination history. Coronavirus exposure in dogs is common. It is an infrequent cause of infectious enteritis in dogs. Infection is highly contagious. Neonatal pups are more severely affected than those of weaning age and adults. Coronavirus is shed in faeces for weeks to months after exposure. Clinical signs of infection can vary but may include acute diarrhoea and vomiting.

TEXT C: _____

History: Epigastric discomfort and persistent nausea

Findings: The pancreas is not well visualised. The gallbladder is thin walled and contains no calculi or sludge. The liver is echogenic, in keeping with steatosis with an echogenic lesion in segment 4 measuring 10mm and a smaller echogenic focus in segment 7 measuring 6mm. Possible small haemangiomata.

The right kidney measures 115mm and is normal in appearance. The left kidney measures 102mm and demonstrates a 12mm mid renal cortical cyst. The spleen span is 86mm. No free fluid.

Conclusion: There is evidence of hepatic steatosis with two echogenic foci, likely reflecting haemangiomata. A repeat ultrasound in 6 months is recommended. No conclusive cause for the patient's symptoms. There is evidence of hepatic steatosis.

TEXT D: _____

Name of Test 1: CALPROTECTIN FAECAL

Clinical Notes: nausea, fatigue

Faecal Calprotectin   H 63   mg/kg   (<50)

Elevated faecal calprotectin indicates a high probability of intestinal inflammation. Levels of faecal calprotectin above 250mg/kg have greater positive predictive value especially in children. For patients with known inflammatory bowel disease in remission, faecal calprotectin above 50mg/kg is associated with an increased risk of relapse over the next 12 months. In patients with faecal calprotectin levels below 50mg/kg with strong clinical indications of intestinal inflammation, a repeat sample may be useful. In small bowel Crohn's, the faecal calprotectin may be within the normal range. Many conditions including bowel cancer, NSAID ulceration, coeliac disease, diverticulitis and chronic inflammation may cause elevated faecal calprotectin. This test has not been validated in children under two years of age.

Name of Test 2: C-REACTIVE PROTEIN

Clinical Notes: fatigue

CRP   7   <1   1   mg/L   (<5)

C-reactive protein (CRP)

Interpretation: Elevation in CRP indicates disease activity of an inflammatory, infective or neoplastic nature. CRP is a more sensitive early indicator of an acute phase response than is the ESR (erythrocyte sedimentation rate) blood test. CRP also returns towards normal more rapidly with improvement or resolution of the disease process.

Decreased CRP values occur when patients are treated with antibiotics containing carboxypenicillins including ticarcillin.

Task 2

Read Texts A-D again and answer Questions 1-15.

Questions 1-6

Decide in which text, A, B, C or D, you can find the information mentioned in Questions 1-6. You may refer to each text more than once. Write your answers in the space provided. An example (0) has been done for you.

> **BOOSTER TIP**
>
> For this task, read the text carefully to locate the **specific information** required for each question. Read the details closely to ensure clear understanding of the text and questions.

In which text can you find information about

0 the recommended daily intake of cheese?

1 a useful prognostic test for intestinal irritation in children over 2 years?

2 the recommended interval until a repeat procedure should be conducted?

3 a possible limitation in accuracy due to the testing procedures used?

4 advising a patient to record their symptoms during a trial?

5 investigating upper abdominal pain and chronic nausea?

6 a disease which can significantly impact the wellbeing of newborn animals?

Write your answers here.

0	1	2	3	4	5	6
A						

Questions 7-10

Answer Questions 7-10 with a word or short phrase from Texts A - D. Each answer may include words, numbers or both.

7 How long should patients follow the baseline diet between the amine challenge and the salicylate challenge?

_____

8 Which organ was unable to be seen clearly in the abdominal ultrasound?

_____

9 What are two common symptoms of gastroenteritis in dogs?

_____ and _____

10 What reactions may occur as a result of sensitivity to amines?

_____

Questions 11-15

Complete Questions 11-15 by using a word or short phrase from Texts A-D. Each answer may include words, numbers or both.

11 Treatment with an extended-spectrum _____ may reduce clinically active inflammation.

12 This procedure may not identify all _____ of the specified infectious agents being screened for.

13 Three conditions which may cause higher levels of faecal calprotectin are _____, _____ and _____.

14 A mid renal cortical cyst found in the left kidney during ultrasound examination was reported to measure _____ mm.

15 Risk indicators for relapse for patients with a history of inflammatory bowel disease include a calprotectin reading of higher than _____.

VOCABULARY PRACTICE 1A: MATCHING MEANING

The words and phrases in Column A appear in Text A, B, C or D. Choose the most suitable word or phrase from Column B for each word or phrase in Column A. Write your answers in the space provided. An example (0) has been done for you.

COLUMN A	COLUMN B
0 **predictive**	A to remove, get rid of something
1 echogenic	B development of painful sores on or in body
2 conclusive	C predisposed
3 remission	D **indicating future probability**
4 methodology	E increased to a higher level
5 reaction	F when signs of a serious illness have reduced and are no longer affecting patient
6 validate	G a standardised procedure
7 ulceration	H definite
8 elevated	I to endorse something based on accurate evidence
9 eliminate	J a response to a stimulus
10 susceptible	K able to reflect sound wave signals

Write your answers here.

0	1	2	3	4	5	6	7	8	9	10
D										

VOCABULARY PRACTICE 1B: COMPLETE THE SENTENCE

Choose the most suitable word from the box to complete each sentence. There is one extra word that you do not need to use. An example (0) has been done for you.

| **remission** | methodology | reaction | conclusive | susceptible |
| ulceration | eliminate | validated | elevated | echogenic |

0   Cancer patients no longer displaying signs after completing treatment are said to be in **remission**.

1   Standardised _____ is used in research testing when investigating diseases.

2   _____ properties of organs help to identify abnormalities in ultrasound exams.

3   The results were _____ by the senior pathologist before being released.

4   All travellers arriving at the airport were screened for _____ temperatures.

5   The patient was advised to _____ peanuts from her diet after experiencing a strong _____ to them on two occasions.

6   Further investigations were scheduled after initial test results offered no _____ findings.

7   Excess acid production may exacerbate _____ of the stomach lining.

READING 2

Read the following text about a clinical placement and answer Questions 1-5.

<u>Placement information for student nurses</u>

Welcome to the Endoscopy Unit at Metropolitan Day Procedure and Specialist Centre.

We look forward to working with you and encourage you to take full advantage of this experience to apply the theory and practical skills you have learned in the classroom to a real-life healthcare setting.

YOU HAVE BEEN PLACED WITH THE GASTROSCOPY TEAM.
YOUR NURSING SUPERVISOR IS KYLA HAMILTON.

<u>Clinical skills development</u>

Under supervision, you will practise admitting patients to the Unit. This will involve asking the patient medical and health questions, explaining what will happen over the course of the day and answering any questions the patient may have.

You will record patient observations and assist with patient care during the pre-, peri- and post-procedure stages and support staff to ensure patients are ready for discharge.

While your placement will primarily focus on your responsibilities within the Gastroscopy team, you will be able to meet and observe a broad range of healthcare professionals working in associated specialist areas. These will include respiratory, gastrointestinal and liver consultants, upper gastrointestinal and colorectal surgeons, anaesthetists, registered nurses, healthcare assistants, scope technicians and the decontamination team.

During your placement with us, there will be many optional learning activities available for you to participate in. You may choose to:

- view colonoscopy, flexible sigmoidoscopy and bronchoscopy procedures.
- shadow the decontamination team for a day and observe how the scopes are sterilised and maintained.
- learn how to use topical anaesthetics such as throat sprays.
- train in collecting biopsy samples.

Your nursing supervisor will oversee your placement, including your attendance at the centre, the achievement of your goals and your interaction with healthcare staff and patients.

It is your responsibility to meet with your nursing supervisor each week to discuss:

- your rostered hours of work with the Gastroscopy team.
- your participation in additional learning opportunities within the Endoscopy Unit.
- your feedback and questions about your placement experience.
- assessment of your clinical practice.

Questions 1-5

For Questions 1-5, decide whether the statements are true (T) or false (F). An example (0) has been done for you.

During their placement with the Endoscopy Unit, student nurses:

0	are assigned to a supervisor.	**T**	F
1	can assist with patient admission and discharge procedures.	T	F
2	are restricted to interaction only with the Gastroscopy team.	T	F
3	are required to observe bronchoscopy and colonoscopy procedures.	T	F
4	are responsible for cleaning the scopes for the decontamination team.	T	F
5	are evaluated by their supervisor.	T	F

VOCABULARY PRACTICE 2: ERROR CORRECTION

Read the following sentences. Look at the prepositions in bold. Some sentences are correct and some contain incorrect prepositions. If a sentence is correct, put a tick (✔) in the space provided at the end of the line. If a sentence is incorrect, write the correct preposition in the space provided at the end of the line. Two examples, (00) and (0), have been done for you.

00	After consultation with an emergency doctor, the patient was admitted **to** the local hospital.	✔
0	Ask the supervisor if you have any questions **to** your clinical placement.	**about**
1	Assessment **of** the course learning objectives is ongoing.	
2	Unlimited access to the student portal ensures you can take full advantage **on** online training materials.	
3	During the course, you will be trained **of** reassuring anxious patients.	
4	Staff are required to participate **in** all workplace hygiene seminars.	
5	Nursing supervisors are expected to apply strong leadership skills **to** the role.	
6	How do you measure achievement **of** your goals?	
7	The patient is looking forward **for** being discharged.	
8	Patients should be advised if their prescribed medication might interact **with** certain foods in their daily diet.	

READING 3: COMPLETE THE SENTENCE

Read the following text about gastroscopy. Choose the best word or phrase (A-I) to complete each sentence 1-8. Write your answers in the space provided. An example (0) has been done for you.

> **BOOSTER TIP**
>
> For this task, look carefully at both the meaning and the structure of the text to ensure it is cohesive and grammatically accurate.

General information for gastroscopy placements

Please familiarise yourself with the following information prior to your placement.

Gastroscopy, or upper endoscopy, is a **(0) minimally invasive medical procedure** that allows a doctor to directly view the upper part of the gastrointestinal tract, (1) _____ , stomach and duodenum.

The instrument used for this procedure is a gastroscope (a thin, flexible tube (2) _____ and a video camera at the other) which enters through the mouth. The (3) _____ and transmitted to a monitor and viewed by the doctor. This allows the diagnosis and treatment of certain conditions without the need for major surgery.

Gastroscopy assists the doctor to evaluate symptoms of persistent upper abdominal pain, nausea, indigestion, repeated vomiting, difficulty swallowing, weight loss, anaemia or bleeding from the upper gastrointestinal tract. It can be used to (4) _____ such as coeliac disease and Barrett's oesophagus. The gastroscope can also be used to (5) _____, including:

- treating bleeding (6) _____ or gastric bleeding
- widening a narrow oesophagus, known as dilatation
- (7) _____ (polypectomy)
- obtaining tissue samples (biopsies)
- removing stones from the bile duct
- placing (8) _____
- locating and removing tumours and foreign objects from the digestive tract.

A **minimally invasive medical procedure**
B removing polyps
C with a lens at one end
D perform simple procedures
E monitor existing conditions
F which includes the oesophagus
G ulcers
H stents through blockages
I images obtained are magnified

Write your answers here.

0	1	2	3	4	5	6	7	8
A								

VOCABULARY PRACTICE 3: WORD FORMATION

Read the following Patient Information Leaflet. Write the correct form of the word given in bold to complete each sentence. You may need to check the words in a dictionary if you are unsure of the appropriate verb, noun, adjective or adverb form to use. An example (0) has been done for you.

POSSIBLE COMPLICATIONS OF UPPER GASTROINTESTINAL ENDOSCOPY		
Upper endoscopy/Gastroscopy is a **(0) commonly** performed and generally safe procedure. Despite this, complications do very occasionally occur and may include:	**(0)**	**common**
Haemorrhage (bleeding): This can occur at a biopsy site or at the site where a polyp has been removed. It is usually minimal and can be (1) _____ through the endoscope. Surgery is rarely required to stop bleeding.	(1)	control
(2) _____ : A tear through the wall of the oesophagus, stomach or duodenum is an (3) _____, but serious complication which may require surgery and carries a risk of (4) _____ .	(2) (3) (4)	perforate common infect
Aspiration pneumonia: This is a rare complication that may occur with (5) _____ of any remaining stomach contents during the (6) _____.	(5) (6)	inhale proceed
Dental: Damage to teeth or the inside of the mouth is rare. Please inform the surgeon if you have dentures, crowns or any (7) _____ teeth which require special care during the endoscopy.	(7)	stable
Anaesthetic: Some patients may have a reaction to the (8) _____ .	(8)	sedate
If problems occur: Complications following upper endoscopy are not common. However, it is important to recognise early signs. Complications are best assessed at the hospital and not over the telephone. Please present to hospital if you develop (9) _____ swallowing, a fever or increasing throat, chest or (10) _____ pain.	(9) (10)	difficult abdomen

Discussion

1. What aspects of a clinical placement do you think are the most useful?
2. How would you explain gastroscopy to a patient?
3. What would you say to a patient who is concerned about possible complications of gastroscopy?

STUDY BOOST 2: WRITING

Organising a medical letter

The information contained in a medical letter should be communicated in a clear and logical way. Organising the content of the letter into sections and paragraphs will help to create a well-structured letter. This will assist the reader to locate key information.

A medical letter may include:

- **Address**

> Morningtown General Practice Clinic
> 53 Petrie Street
> Morningtown

- **Date**

> 14 October 2020
> 14/10/2020
> 14/10/20
> 14.10.20

- **Opening salutation**

If you do not know the name of the person you are writing to, use:	If you know the name of the person you are writing to, use:
To whom it may concern	Dear Dr Vescovi
	Dear Mr Forbes

- **Reference to whom or what the letter is about**

Tell the reader who or what the letter is about.

> Re: Mr David O'Connor DOB: 16/11/1965

- **Introduction**

Introduce or refer to the patient.

State the reason for the correspondence.

> Thank you for referring Mr David O'Connor. I met with Mr O'Connor on 22/03/20__ to discuss his ongoing symptoms.

- **Body**

The body is made up of a number of paragraphs. Two or three paragraphs are usually sufficient. One main topic per paragraph helps to keep the message clear. The information included in the body of the letter will vary according to the task.

Organising paragraphs according to topic, for example, relevant patient history, tests performed, current medications, treatment, recommendations or future action required will help you to structure your letter effectively.

TEST PERFORMED

Following consultation, Mr O'Connor underwent gastroscopy which revealed small intestinal bacterial overgrowth (SIBO).

PRESCRIBED TREATMENT

I have prescribed a course of cycling antibiotics to treat SIBO. I have directed him to take Keflex for one 24-tablet course plus one repeat, then have a two week break from antibiotics. He is then to take Noroxin for two weeks followed by a further two-week break. Lastly, he should take Flagyl for two weeks. Cycling these antibiotics over a period of time should minimise any risks of triggering problems with resistant organisms.

FUTURE ACTION

I have instructed him to make an appointment to see me should his symptoms recur.

It may be useful to organise your letter chronologically. Sometimes, dates of tests and other important events will assist you with the organisation of your letter. Begin with the earliest relevant events and finish with the most recent information.

Look at how chronological order is used in these examples.

✗	✓
*I performed gastroscopy on **13 April 20__** and found no evidence of coeliac disease, gastritis or reflux.* *I consulted with Mr O'Connor on **22 March 20__** and discussed a number of issues, including his ongoing intermittent nausea and the results of investigations performed to date.*	*I consulted with Mr O'Connor on **22 March 20__** and discussed a number of issues, including his ongoing intermittent nausea and the results of investigations performed to date.* *I performed gastroscopy on **13 April 20__** and found no evidence of coeliac disease, gastritis or reflux.*

- **Conclusion**

    Give final remarks.

    Make a polite statement to offer the reader further information if required.

> *I have recommended that Mr O'Connor should see a dietician for advice on improving his overall digestive function. Please do contact me if you require any further information regarding this treatment plan.*

- **Complimentary close**

If you do not know the name of the person you are writing to, use:	If you know the name of the person you are writing to, use:
Yours faithfully	*Yours sincerely*
Dr Paul Murphy	*Dr Paul Murphy*

WRITING PRACTICE 1

Look at the Letter of Referral below which has been separated into sections A-I.

Choose the most suitable heading from the list in the box below for each section of the letter (A-I) and write the heading in the space provided. The first one has been done for you.

HEADINGS
- INTRODUCTION
- DATE
- BODY - TREATMENT
- OPENING SALUTATION
- COMPLIMENTARY CLOSE
- **ADDRESS**
- CONCLUSION
- REFERENCE TO WHOM OR WHAT THE LETTER IS ABOUT
- BODY - INVESTIGATIONS PERFORMED

Letter of Referral

A   ADDRESS

Dr Saldanha
Southside Pet Emergency Hospital
Brooktown

B

23 May 20__

C

Dear Dr Saldanha

D

Re: GEORGE, male labradoodle, 18 months

E

George requires specialist assessment and intensive monitoring of his ongoing symptoms. George, an 18-month-old labradoodle who weighs 20kg, presented to my clinic on 22 May 20__ with a 12-hour history of vomiting and diarrhoea. On presentation, George had significant abdominal pain and was moderately dehydrated.

F

Blood tests conducted were unremarkable (mild elevation of GGT) as was abdominal radiography. No obvious or bony object was seen and there was no significant gas accumulation pattern that suggests obstruction.

G

George was given an antiemetic injection (metoclopramide) and tramadol (80mg) was administered for pain relief. He remained under observation for 24 hours but his condition has continued to deteriorate.

H

I have discussed George's need for specialist care with his owner, Rebecca Sullivan, and have confirmed that I am referring George to you. Please do not hesitate to contact me if you require additional information.

I

Yours sincerely
Dr Lin Choi
Veterinarian

WRITING PRACTICE 2

Read the Letter of Referral again and answer Questions 1-9.

Decide in which section of the Letter of Referral (A-I) you can find the information mentioned in Questions 1-9. You may refer to each section more than once. Write your answers in the space provided. An example (0) has been done for you.

Which section (A-I) contains a phrase or sentence which:

0   shows the name and job title of the referring doctor?
1   offers to provide further details if required?
2   provides the location of the specialist doctor's practice?
3   states the reason for referral of the patient?
4   mentions consultation with the owner?
5   gives the findings of an investigation?
6   provides identification details of the patient?
7   refers to the duration of the patient's symptoms prior to consultation?
8   describes treatment administered to the patient?
9   describes the initial condition of the patient?

Write your answers here.

0	1	2	3	4	5	6	7	8	9
I									

WRITING PRACTICE 3

Letter of Discharge

Complete the Letter of Discharge using sentences A-J. Write your answers in the space provided. An example (0) has been done for you.

35 Tilby Avenue
Sunny Bay

27 May 20__

Dear Ms Sullivan

RE: George 26/01/20___

George was referred to Southside Pet Emergency Hospital by your regular vet due to a recent history of vomiting, diarrhoea, lethargy and decreased appetite. **(0)** <u>He is now ready for discharge</u>.

Prior to admission at Southside Pet Emergency Hospital, George underwent several blood tests and an abdominal radiograph was performed. (1) _____
_____

On presentation at Southside Pet Emergency Hospital, George was moderately dehydrated and also had some abdominal pain. (2) _____
_____

Whilst in hospital, George has been monitored intensively and has received supportive care to aid his recovery, including intravenous fluids to maintain hydration and organ perfusion, pain relief, probiotics and gastro-protectants. (3) _____

He has responded well to this treatment and is continuing to regain his appetite. However, he regurgitated twice in hospital last night, leading us to believe he may not be completely over his illness.

(4) _____
_____

As such, we are happy to discharge him into your care.

Regarding medications, please give Protexin (probiotic), 3g, ONCE a day, orally, for the next 4 days. (5) _____

Please feed him a bland, highly digestible diet for the next 3 days. (6) _____
_____ Start with small meals 3-4 times per day, then gradually increase the amount of food given over 2-3 days. Gradually transition over 3-5 days back to George's normal diet.

(7) _____
_____
_____ If any of these signs appear, please seek veterinary advice immediately from your primary care vet or return to Southside Pet Emergency Hospital.

If possible, collect a stool sample from George using the container provided and deliver to your vet for testing. (8) _____

Please make an appointment in 2-3 days with your regular veterinarian for a check-up.

(9) _____
_____

Yours sincerely
Dr Pree Saldanha

UNIT 6 GASTROINTESTINAL INVESTIGATIONS

A Today George is comfortable, has eaten well and has had no further vomiting since this morning.

B **He is now ready for discharge.**

C This may reveal the cause of George's illness.

D In order to further investigate his clinical signs, a specialist ultrasound was performed, the findings of which were consistent with gastroenteritis.

E If you have any further concerns or questions, please do not hesitate to contact Southside Pet Emergency Hospital or George's regular vet.

F These did not reveal any significant abnormalities which could be responsible for his clinical signs.

G Boiled chicken and rice is a good option.

H Monitor for a return of clinical signs which may include vomiting, lethargy, inappetence, increasing amounts or persistent diarrhoea and abdominal discomfort.

I In addition, he has been given anti-nausea injections daily.

J The next dose is due tomorrow morning.

Write your answers here.

0	1	2	3	4	5	6	7	8	9
B									

UNIT 7 | INFECTION PREVENTION AND CONTROL

STUDY FOCUS

Reading: Identifying main ideas, locating specific information and recognising attitude, opinion and pronoun references

Vocabulary: Preventing and controlling the spread of infection

Speaking: Managing the structure of discourse in a consultation

Exploring the topic

In pairs or groups, discuss the following questions.

- What is infection prevention and control?
- Why is infection prevention and control important?
- What are some infection prevention and control strategies that you are familiar with?

STUDY BOOST 1: READING AND VOCABULARY

READING 1

Read the excerpts from research articles relating to infection prevention and control. For Questions 1-6, choose the most suitable answer A, B or C. An example (0) has been done for you.

> **BOOSTER TIP**
>
> For this task, look closely at the words and expressions used to convey information presented to the reader as fact, attitude or opinion.

0 In this paragraph, the writer suggests that

A junior staff must mentor senior staff to ensure that they comply with infection control practices.

B <u>adherence to infection control policies is the responsibility of everybody in the workplace.</u>

C reporting breaches of infection control procedures results in higher rates of compliance.

> Jennifer Zhao, a nurse mentor from Westlake University Hospital, encourages nursing students under **her** supervision to report breaches of infection control measures. 'I understand that it may be difficult for a trainee nurse to report on a senior nurse. It is essential for all staff at all times to comply with infection prevention and control procedures. Lapses in infection prevention and control practices will be reported to the Infection Control Team.'

1 What point does Dr Tseng make about hand hygiene procedures?
   A Washing your hands after removing single-use gloves is not necessary.
   B The transmission of Gram-negative bacteria is not affected by hand hygiene measures.
   C Simple hand hygiene measures can determine the success of infection prevention and control in certain settings.

According to Dr Martin Tseng, a neonatologist with 40 years of experience, many of the everyday infection control practices **that** have become standard for healthcare workers are actually just common sense. 'Washing your hands before and after handling each baby, wearing single-use gloves when changing a nappy and washing your hands after removing your gloves are essential to reduce the risk of spread of infectious agents,' explains Dr Tseng.

'I can recall numerous cases in neonatal units where cross-transmission of Gram-negative bacteria occurred and babies died as a result. In many of these cases, levels of hand hygiene compliance were found to be low. It's devastating to think these deaths were most likely preventable and may have occurred simply because somebody didn't wash their hands.'

2 The author uses an example to illustrate that
   A it is not always fully understood how a blood-borne disease has been transmitted.
   B transmission of a blood-borne disease can only occur when there is direct contact between patients.
   C there is a high risk of blood-borne disease transmission during oral surgery.

Patients with blood-borne viral infections such as hepatitis B, hepatitis C and HIV can be treated safely and effectively in dental health care settings when standard infection control practices are followed. Patient-to-patient transmission of blood-borne pathogens is not common, but cases have been recorded.

In one case of patient-to-patient transmission investigated by Dr Christian Faulkner, a patient contracted hepatitis B while undergoing oral surgery. The source of transmission in this instance was determined to be a patient infected with hepatitis B who had undergone the extraction of several teeth earlier in the day. The two patients had had no direct contact with each other and investigators reported good adherence to infection control procedures by the staff in this practice. In the absence of a clear link between the two cases, Dr Faulkner reported that **his** team could only speculate that the virus had remained on a surface which had been contaminated with spots or drops of blood, which then spread to the patient. No other patients and no staff members were affected.

3 Dr Adelina Kowalski's research concluded that
   A staff should attend regular training to better understand the importance of hand hygiene measures in the workplace.
   B there are a number of reasons why staff may not always comply with hand hygiene practices.
   C frequent hand washing is not necessary when staff are very busy.

Low compliance of hand hygiene practices is not always due to laziness or forgetfulness. In a recent study, Dr Adelina Kowalski investigated attitudes towards infection prevention and control protocols. She formed the view that when senior staff considered frequent hand washing to be an unnecessary burden on their already heavy workload, **this** resulted in low rates of hand hygiene compliance among all staff. The issue of low and non-compliance with regards to hand hygiene is actually complex. It is important to develop a deeper understanding of workplace culture to identify and overcome barriers to effective infection prevention and control practices.

4   Dr Amy Arthy's clinical experience has informed her opinion that
    A   surgical site infection following caesarean section is difficult to avoid.
    B   obstetricians must provide better mental health support for new mothers.
    C   increased patient education about post-surgical infection may result in improved outcomes.

> One aspect of patient-centred healthcare is providing patients with clear and consistent communication relating to the specific risks associated with their treatment. Obstetrician Dr Amy Arthy has managed multiple cases where a lack of patient education around wound care has contributed to the development of a surgical site infection.
>
> 'We need to be vigilant about having conversations with surgical patients, explicitly outlining wound care and how to spot signs of infection,' Dr Arthy insists. 'We have to repeat these conversations while in hospital and provide written materials for patients to refer to after discharge. **I** recently saw a patient, whose baby had been delivered via caesarean section, on the 11th postoperative day for a maternal wellbeing check. The patient had developed cellulitis, and an intense, red rash had spread from the surgical wound across her lower and upper abdomen, upper thighs and back. Whilst this patient's cellulitis resolved with oral antibiotics, her abdomen was tender and sore and she reported that it was painful to hold and feed her new baby. Even though this was considered to be an uncomplicated case of cellulitis, it was a barrier to her wellbeing and also to her recovery. This patient may have sought medical advice sooner if she had been more alert to the signs of infection.'

5   Why does the writer specifically mention dementia patients?
    A   To suggest that uncooperative patients should be placed in isolation.
    B   To highlight that patients with dementia face increased challenges when placed in isolation.
    C   To argue that nursing interventions are not beneficial for patients with dementia in isolation.

> Identifying and managing infection risk by limiting exposure to infectious agents is an integral aspect of patient safety and quality care. Restricting the movement of residents or confining them to their rooms may be necessary during the outbreak of an infectious disease.
>
> Patients with dementia who are placed in isolation may experience more frequent episodes of delirium as well as increased levels of anxiety, agitation and hostility. **They** may be uncooperative and may not fully comply with requests.
>
> Nursing management may include allocating specific staff to an affected resident, placing the affected resident in an isolation room close to staff, providing reassurance, frequent intervention with diversional therapy and surrounding the resident with familiar items which can be cleaned or discarded when the outbreak has ended.

6   Dr Lewis believes that
    A the method of instruction is not important to the success of infection control training.
    B in-person role play supports the best learning strategies in infection control training.
    C online education offers the most valuable training in infection control.

> Efforts must be made to contain any infectious disease that has the potential to cause significant illness or an outbreak.
>
> General guidelines for managing infection prevention and control, together with the risk assessment of individual healthcare workplaces, inform decisions on procedures to be implemented to protect the health of patients, visitors and staff.
>
> According to Dr Eric Lewis, an infection and control consultant, clinical preparation, incorporating regular in-house training for all staff to consolidate **their** knowledge of workplace procedures, is integral to the success of any infection control program irrespective of the healthcare setting.
>
> Dr Lewis strongly advocates that staff training, including rehearsals of individual roles should be based on realistic scenarios and must be completed to a level where staff can recognise and implement the relevant procedures without hesitation when a risk is identified.
>
> Participating in simulated activities in face-to-face group training sessions allows staff to discover how they might respond to real-life situations, while demonstrating the skills required to manage any risks. It also provides trainers with the opportunity to give immediate feedback, offer suggestions for alternative responses and address any issues they may have observed during the role play. 'In my experience, this practical approach to training is much more effective than theory-based learning or completing online courses,' says Dr Lewis. 'Being able to adapt responses and manage unforeseen circumstances is part of successful infection control.'

VOCABULARY PRACTICE 1A: MATCHING REFERENCE PRONOUNS

Read through Texts 0-6 again. Look at the underlined pronouns in bold in each text. Match each pronoun listed in Column A with the word or expression it refers to in Column B. Write your answers in the space provided. An example (0) has been done for you.

READING TEXT	COLUMN A		COLUMN B
0	**her**	A	infection control practices
1	that	B	an extra burden on a heavy workload
2	his	C	Dr Amy Arthy
3	this	D	all staff
4	I	**E**	**nurse mentor**
5	they	F	Dr Faulkner
6	their	G	patients with dementia

Write your answers here.

0	1	2	3	4	5	6
E						

VOCABULARY PRACTICE 1B: WORD FORMS

Look carefully at the text relating to chickenpox. Choose the most suitable option A, B or C to complete each sentence. Write your answers in the space provided. An example (0) has been done for you.

Chickenpox, caused by the varicella-zoster virus, is highly **(0) infectious.**

The characteristic itchy rash (1) _____ with chickenpox develops into blisters which dry into scabs and becomes visible 10-21 days after (2) _____ to the virus.

Chickenpox is easily (3) _____, particularly among children, from one infected person to another through airborne droplets produced when sneezing or coughing. This is largely (4) _____ through common infection control strategies, such as hand hygiene, wearing face masks and (5) _____ infected children to ensure they do not have contact with adult family members, young babies, pregnant women or those who are immunocompromised.

(6) _____ with regulations in childcare centres and schools, which clearly state that children with chickenpox must not attend until they no longer present a risk of spreading the infection, also plays a vital part in the control of chickenpox.

The chickenpox vaccine is a relatively recent addition to the childhood immunisation program. While the vaccine has a high rate of success in preventing chickenpox, it is still possible for someone who has been vaccinated to (7) _____ chickenpox, although it will be a much milder form of the virus than for anyone (8) _____.

In the past, and before the chickenpox vaccine became readily available, it was widely believed by the general public that children would suffer mild symptoms of the disease, whereas those who caught chickenpox as an adult were at risk of far more severe consequences.

With this in mind, parents of children with chickenpox would invite children of friends and neighbours to 'chickenpox parties' to visit the infectious child in the hope they too would catch the disease and develop lifetime (9) _____.

Medical advice, however, warns against 'chickenpox parties' as, in a small number of cases, the disease can lead to serious (10) _____ including encephalitis, bacterial skin infections and shingles in later life.

0	A	infection	B	infected	**C**	**infectious**
1	A	associates	B	associated	C	association
2	A	exposure	B	exposed	C	exposes
3	A	transmission	B	transmits	C	transmitted
4	A	preventable	B	unpreventable	C	preventing
5	A	isolated	B	isolation	C	isolating
6	A	Compliant	B	Compliance	C	Non-compliance
7	A	contracted	B	contraction	C	contract
8	A	unvaccinated	B	vaccination	C	vaccinated
9	A	immunised	B	immune	C	immunity
10	A	complicated	B	complications	C	complicates

Write your answers here.

0	1	2	3	4	5	6	7	8	9	10
C										

READING 2

Read the following text about tuberculosis and answer Questions 1-8. Write your answers in the space provided.

> **BOOSTER TIP**
>
> For this task, read the text carefully to identify the information required to answer each question. Read the details closely to ensure clear understanding of the text and questions.

Antibiotic resistance and tuberculosis

Antibiotic resistant organisms are associated with significant morbidity and mortality. Every year, hundreds of thousands of deaths worldwide can be attributed to infections caused by resistant bacteria. These infections are increasingly difficult to treat because bacteria are rapidly becoming resistant to all currently available antibiotics.

According to Professor McDermott, a specialist in infectious diseases, as the world's most infectious disease, tuberculosis is of particular concern. 'Along with malaria and HIV, tuberculosis is also one of the world's deadliest infectious diseases. In fact, prior to the discovery of antibiotics, tuberculosis was one of the leading causes of death globally,' says Professor McDermott. Following the adoption of antibiotic treatment, incidences of tuberculosis declined. However, more recently, there has been a resurgence of cases due to the emergence of drug-resistant strains.

One of the major contributing factors to the increasing incidence of drug-resistant tuberculosis is poor patient compliance with the demanding requirements of treatment. Susceptible tuberculosis responds to the first-line drug therapies rifampicin and isoniazid, which must be taken every day for at least six months to eliminate the bacteria. 'Patients often stop taking the medication when they start feeling better, but an absence of symptoms is not an indication that the infection has resolved,' explains Professor McDermott. Stopping treatment prematurely gives the surviving bacteria the opportunity to mutate into resistant strains, against which antibiotics are notably less effective. If high level resistance occurs against first-line drug therapies, multi-drug resistant tuberculosis can develop. This then requires significantly longer, more complex treatment plans involving second-line drugs with higher levels of toxicity.

One strategy to improve medication adherence, known as directly observed therapy (DOT), is widely used even though it is labour-, time- and resource-intensive. DOT involves a healthcare worker observing the patient taking each dose of medication in person every day for the duration of their treatment. Professor McDermott acknowledges that some patients may perceive the requirement for daily supervision as a lack of confidence in their ability to competently self-administer their medication. Despite **this**, Professor McDermott insists that failure by the healthcare system to consistently monitor individual patients would put the health of the broader community at unacceptable risk.

Professor McDermott is exploring ways of giving tuberculosis patients more control over their treatment, by exploiting existing technology to monitor medication compliance of patients with susceptible tuberculosis, which he hopes will improve medication adherence and help to prevent drug-resistant strains from developing. The main objective is to develop a smartphone application which will improve the patient medication monitoring experience for the patient. It is anticipated that the app will allow patients greater flexibility around the self-administration of their medication and the reporting requirements, which will result in increased willingness to complete the treatment plan. In addition, implementing technology for daily communication between patient and supervisor will provide a 'more efficient and cost-effective option for healthcare services,' says Professor McDermott.

Mobile application developer Nancy Bell is excited to be collaborating on this project with Professor McDermott. She is confident that the application has the potential to transform the patient experience. According to Ms Bell, the most critical feature of the app will be an alarm which prompts users to take their antibiotics at scheduled times. A video recording communication function is also to be included as an integral part of the app to allow users to video themselves taking their medication, which is shared with a healthcare worker responsible for remotely monitoring patient compliance. 'The healthcare worker can intervene if poor compliance is detected and address any social, psychological or emotional issues that might be affecting the patient's ability to adhere to the treatment plan,' explains Ms Bell.

A symptom tracker is being designed as part of the app to encourage users to input any symptoms they experience. This data will be analysed through an algorithm programmed into the app which detects signs of drug resistance and then activates a prompt to encourage patients to seek professional advice regarding their treatment. 'We hope that this feature of the app may play a role in detecting resistant cases sooner, enabling key early intervention,' says Ms Bell.

While Professor McDermott expects the app to meet with widespread approval, he warns that issues associated with using digital technology should be discussed when promoting it to tuberculosis patients. Specifically, in order to use the app, users must have access to a digital device with reliable internet connectivity. A functional level of digital literacy is required to use the app as no training is provided.

Professor McDermott reveals that the fight against tuberculosis is intensifying. 'Cases of extensively drug-resistant tuberculosis, are now being reported in several regions,' says Professor McDermott. He is referring to tuberculosis that has become resistant to the first-line drugs, and to at least one of the second-line drugs. 'As tuberculosis is becoming harder to treat, it is apparent that we need to successfully manage every single case in order to reduce the likelihood of drug-resistant strains developing. To do this, we need new approaches and we need to act quickly to give us the best chance of success.'

1. What information can be found in the first paragraph?
    A. the difference between morbidity and mortality
    B. the degree to which resistant bacteria is impacting global mortality rates
    C. the importance of eliminating antibiotic resistant organisms
    D. the challenge for scientists to develop new strains of antibiotics

2. What point is made about susceptible tuberculosis in paragraph 3?
    A. Antibiotics are equally effective against susceptible and multi-drug resistant tuberculosis.
    B. Patients do not need to continue treatment when signs of the infection disappear.
    C. Patient behaviour can cause drug resistance to occur.
    D. Second-line drug treatments are more effective than first-line therapies.

3. In paragraph 4, it is suggested that DOT is
    A. a costly program to administer.
    B. only useful in limited settings.
    C. most important in the initial stages of treatment.
    D. an efficient approach to disease management.

4 When the writer uses the expression 'Despite this' in paragraph 4, 'this' is referring to
   A patients being unable to manage their treatment independently.
   B the risk of causing an outbreak in the community.
   C the inadequate supervision of individual patients by medical professionals.
   D patient resentment towards the need for daily monitoring.

5 According to paragraph 5, the most important motivation for Professor McDermott's investigation into the development of an app is to
   A completely replace professional healthcare services with technology.
   B instruct patients how to communicate clearly with healthcare professionals.
   C offer patients greater autonomy regarding the management of their treatment.
   D provide a more convenient reporting system for healthcare professionals.

6 Ms Bell explains that the app will
   A alert healthcare staff to users with poor medication compliance.
   B send a reminder to patients if they have not administered their medication on time.
   C inform healthcare staff about patients' personal problems.
   D automatically schedule a medical appointment for patients showing signs of resistance.

7 What should potential users be told about the app?
   A No particular expertise is required by the user.
   B Regular internet access is not essential.
   C Training is available for first-time users.
   D Users must be familiar with digital technology.

8 In the final paragraph, Professor McDermott infers that
   A changes to tuberculosis treatments will not impact drug-resistant tuberculosis.
   B current tuberculosis infection control strategies are failing.
   C new strains of tuberculosis are not a cause for concern.
   D intensive case management is only needed when significant numbers of people are infected.

Write your answers here.

1	2	3	4	5	6	7	8

VOCABULARY PRACTICE 2: SENTENCE COMPLETION

Match the beginning of sentences in Column A with the most suitable ending in Column B. Write your answers in the space provided. An example (0) has been done for you.

COLUMN A	COLUMN B
0 <u>Measles, which is a notifiable disease, is caused by</u>	A to eliminate Mycobacterium, the bacteria which causes tuberculosis.
1 Methicillin-resistant Staphylococcus aureus, which can cause serious infections including septicaemia, is difficult to treat due	B <u>a highly infectious virus.</u>
	C the transmission of bacteria between patients.
	D multi-drug resistant organisms.
2 Artificial intelligence has identified a compound with antimicrobial properties which has demonstrated a remarkable ability	E treat the infection.
	F the condition has resolved.
3 Increasingly, hospitals are moving towards single-room patient accommodation in an effort to limit	G to resistance to some antibiotics.
	H adept at developing resistance.
	I is increasing.
4 Contact precautions should be taken for patients known to be colonised or infected with	
5 Staff with skin and soft tissue infections are to be excluded from clinical duties until	
6 Decisions around treatment must be based on the epidemiology of the organism and the resources that are available to	
7 The incidence of community-acquired Clostridium difficile infections	
8 Gram-negative bacteria, such as E. coli, are particularly	

Write your answers here.

0	1	2	3	4	5	6	7	8
B								

READING 3: COMPLETE THE SENTENCE

Read the following text about face masks. Choose the best phrase (A-K) to complete each sentence 1-10. Write your answers in the space provided. An example (0) has been done for you.

BOOSTER TIP
For this task, look carefully at both the meaning and the structure of the text to ensure it is cohesive and grammatically accurate.

Face masks

Healthcare facilities are responsible for establishing and maintaining stringent workplace protocols **(0) <u>which provide staff and patients with a safe environment</u>** and manage the risk of nosocomial transmission and exposure to biological hazards.

When visiting healthcare premises, (1) _____ dental surgeries, patients expect to be surrounded by sanitised surfaces, to have access to soap or sanitiser to clean their hands and to (2) _____ personal protection equipment (PPE), which could include disposable gloves, gowns, head coverings, eye protection and face masks.

During the COVID-19 pandemic, many health authorities around the world mandated the wearing of face masks (3) _____ in an attempt to limit the potential spread of the COVID-19 virus throughout the community. For many people, this requirement was adopted without hesitation. (4) _____ to comply with it.

Concerns that were raised about wearing a face mask could be characterised into three main areas. The (5) _____ wearing a face mask could effectively prevent the spread of infectious diseases, (6) _____, among the community.

The second was the reported physical discomfort of wearing a face mask, while the third indicated (7) _____ open face-to-face communication.

While experts generally agree that specialised and disposable face masks provide (8) _____ the spread of respiratory droplets, they do also say that any mask that covers the nose and mouth is useful.

Common complaints associated with the discomfort of wearing masks included the sensation of being unable to breathe as easily as usual and of producing unclear, barely audible speech. Many people also expressed frustration at not being able to see facial expressions (9) _____ that they have understood the message accurately.

Improving the comfort and look of face masks led to the emergence of a new and increasingly popular trend of people producing home-made washable fabric masks with adjustable straps in colours and styles which reflected their personalities.

Creatively customised mask designs depicted cartoon characters, movie icons, or facial expressions, such as a smiling mouth.

Some face masks were designed with a transparent mouth section to (10) _____. This feature was particularly appreciated by those with hearing loss who were dependent on lip-reading spoken words for successful communication.

A such as respiratory illnesses
B Others expressed reluctance
C **which provide staff and patients with a safe environment**
D facilitate more natural communication
E such as hospitals, medical clinics and
F anxiety about its impediment to clear and
G be attended by medical staff wearing appropriate
H which they often rely on to check
I first questioned whether
J by the general public when outside of their home
K the most effective barrier to

Write your answers here.

0	1	2	3	4	5	6	7	8	9	10
C										

STUDY BOOST 2: SPEAKING
Managing the structure of discourse in a consultation

1 Exploring the use of cohesive devices

The appropriate use of cohesive devices enables the healthcare professional to communicate in a clear and organised way and facilitates better understanding by the patient.

Cohesive devices help you to:
- make logical connections between ideas
- place actions or events in the correct order
- avoid unnecessary repetition of words or phrases
- extend your responses and explanations.

Compare the two conversations. Conversation 1 has been written **without** cohesive devices and Conversation 2 has been written **with** cohesive devices. Notice how **cohesive devices** have been used in Conversation 2 to facilitate clear and organised communication.

SETTING: A sick boy and his parent are visiting a general practice medical clinic. The physician is concluding the consultation.

Conversation 1: **without** cohesive devices	Conversation 2: **with** cohesive devices
Physician: So, over the past 24 hours, your son has had a fever with chills and pain on swallowing, swollen glands and has been feeling faint. Have I missed anything?	**Physician:** So, **to sum up**, over the past 24 hours, your son has had a fever with chills, pain on swallowing, swollen glands and has been feeling faint. Have I missed anything?
Parent: No, that's everything. Do you know what could be wrong?	**Parent:** No, that's everything. Do you know what could be wrong?
Physician: He has a severe infection. We need to find out what it is. When we find out what it is, we can treat him.	**Physician:** He has a severe infection **and** we need to find out what it is **so** we can treat him.
Parent: Is it serious?	**Parent:** Is it serious?
Physician: He needs hospital treatment. He is very unwell. I'm going to call the hospital and tell them you are coming via private transport. I'm going to send through a written referral marked 'urgent' to the hospital. You won't have any delays on arrival. His illness is severe. He needs to be placed in isolation. If you drive him to hospital yourself, it is important that you go there directly. Don't make any stops on the way. I can organise an ambulance if you prefer.	**Physician:** He needs hospital treatment **because** he is very unwell. **Firstly**, I'm going to call the hospital and tell them you are coming via private transport. I'm **also** going to send through a written referral marked 'urgent' to the hospital **so** you won't have any delays on arrival. Your son needs to be placed in isolation **due to** the nature and severity of his illness. If you drive him to hospital yourself, it is **particularly** important that you go there directly. Don't make any stops on the way. **Alternatively**, I can organise an ambulance if you prefer.

2 Examples of cohesive devices to develop clear and organised communication

Adding	and also as well as in addition to besides	- After surgery, it is important to breathe deeply **and** cough against a firm pillow to help your lungs to fully inflate. This helps to prevent post surgical complications such as pneumonia. - Sulfasalazine is a medicine used to treat rheumatoid arthritis. It can **also** be used to treat other diseases such as ulcerative colitis. - Strengthening **as well as** stretching exercises can help with lower back pain. - **In addition to** seeing your physician for an annual skin exam, you should check your own skin for any changes. - **Besides** the question about your asthma medication, is there anything else you would like to ask me?
Cause and effect	because because of as a result as a result of therefore due to so	- Antibiotics administered intravenously act quickly on the body **because** the drugs are delivered directly into the bloodstream. - Hygiene measures have been increased in the nursing home **because of** the current gastroenteritis outbreak. - You have sustained a partial thickness burn to your left hand. **As a result**, you will require a skin graft to assist healing and minimise scarring. - Joint problems in dogs can occur **as a result of** excess weight. - Your test results were inconclusive; **therefore**, we need to investigate further. - Hearing loss is treatable **due to** technological advances in hearing aids. - Your pulse is irregular **so** we would like to keep you here for observation.
Contrasting	whereas unlike however alternatively but	- Oropharyngeal dysphagia is typically caused by a neurological problem, **whereas** esophageal dysphagia is usually the result of a blockage or irritation. - **Unlike** compression stockings, anti-embolic stockings are not suitable for the treatment or management of venous disease. - Plaque can be removed by gentle brushing. **However**, calculus can only be removed by a dental professional. - Please come to the clinic every day to have your dressing changed. **Alternatively**, we can arrange a community nurse to visit you at home. - You need to avoid eating dairy products for 2 weeks, **but** you can include dairy substitutes in your diet.

Emphasising	significantly above all especially particularly	• Your dog's teeth have **significantly** more tartar on them now than when I saw him this time last year. • **Above all**, the wound must be kept dry for the next 48 hours. Moisture slows the healing process. • Regular glaucoma screening is **especially** important after the age of 40. • Signs of Sever's disease include heel pain during physical exercise, **particularly** activities which involve running or jumping.
Giving good and bad news	fortunately unfortunately	• **Fortunately**, cataract surgery generally has very good outcomes. • **Unfortunately**, part of your toenail will have to be removed to prevent infection.
Illustrating	such as for example for instance includes including	• If you notice your 12-month-old is not meeting milestones, **such as** picking up small objects or babbling, please contact your physician. • Treating late-stage metastatic cancer, **for example** malignant melanoma that has spread to distant organs, can be difficult. • Treatment for cancer **includes** chemotherapy, radiation and surgery. • Prenatal vitamins, **including** folic acid and iron, support the healthy development of your baby.
Introducing new information	by the way incidentally	• **By the way**, you are due for a pap smear. Do you want it done now? • **Incidentally**, it is a good idea at your age to start having annual physical exams.
Sequencing	first first of all next after that last of all before after	• To use a blood pressure monitor, **first** you need to sit quietly in a comfortable chair for about 5 minutes. • **First of all**, I am going to ask you some questions about your most recent illness. • **Next**, I am going to ask about your family's medical history. • **After that**, I am going to examine you. • **Last of all**, I am going to give you a medical certificate because you will not be fit to return to work for at least another week. • **Before** a blood transfusion is given, the blood group of both the donor and the recipient must be known. • **After** donating blood, drink plenty of fluids, eat a nutritious meal and avoid strenuous exercise for at least 12 hours.

Restating key points	in other words to sum up to summarise	• I would like you to follow a low residue diet. **In other words**, avoid raw fruit and vegetables, high fibre foods and all foods with pips or skins. • **To sum up**, you don't have an autoimmune disease, but I would like you to have a blood test to make sure we are not missing anything. • So, **to summarise**, you have sharp, stabbing pains in your left kneecap which is most noticeable when you walk up and down stairs. Is that correct?
Qualification	even so all the same having said that	• You do not have any signs of autoimmune disease. **Even so**, it is best that we rule it out with a blood test. • I am fairly certain your symptoms will resolve on their own. **All the same**, I would like to see you again in a week. • You are younger than the usual age to have your prostate checked. **Having said that**, you have some unusual symptoms, so I think you should be examined.

SPEAKING PRACTICE 1A: COMPLETE THE SENTENCE

For Questions 1-10, choose the most suitable answer A, B, or C to complete each sentence. An example (0) has been done for you.

0   We wear medical scrubs _____ they are hygienic, microbial and comfortable.

    A   therefore   B   due to   **C   because**

1   Symptoms such as nausea and headaches may be _____ stress rather than an infection.

    A   due to   B   including   C   as a result

2   So, _____, you are worried that your incision may be infected because you have had some sharp pains around the site and you feel nauseous.

    A   fortunately   B   such as   C   to summarise

3   Hydroxychloroquine can be used to treat parasitic infections. _____, it is not routinely used to treat parasitic infections these days because of resistance by the parasites.

    A   Alternatively   B   Having said that   C   After that

4   If left untreated, haemochromatosis can lead to a number of complications, _____ in the joints, heart, liver and pancreas.

    A   includes   B   especially   C   as well as

5   Swimming, _____ running, places very little pressure on your joints and is an excellent choice of exercise for people who find high impact exercise too strenuous.

    A   above all   B   therefore   C   unlike

6 I suspect you have a urinary tract infection. _____, we need to do a urinalysis.

   A   First of all   B   In addition to   C   For instance

7 Your breathing is laboured _____ your airways are inflamed.

   A   due to   B   because   C   as a result of

8 Changing positions during labour, _____ walking, rocking, squatting and using a birthing ball, can help to manage the pain of contractions.

   A   even so   B   for example   C   by the way

9 _____, you won't be able to have surgery for six months if you have a cortisone injection to relieve the pain in your shoulder.

   A   Particularly   B   Whereas   C   Incidentally

10 The swelling around the eye appears to be the result of an allergic reaction. _____, an infection of the eye can be very serious, so I am prescribing a course of antibiotics as a precaution.

   A   However   B   For instance   C   Particularly

SPEAKING PRACTICE 1B: MULTIPLE CHOICE CLOZE

School nurse Sophie Jones recently posted the following message to the school's social media site.

For Questions 1-10, choose the most suitable answer A, B, or C to complete each sentence. An example (0) has been done for you.

Hello, everyone. There are several cases of head lice in the school at the moment, so I am here to give you a quick reminder of what to do if you discover your child has head lice. **(0) First**, closely inspect the hair and scalp for signs of infestation. If you notice live lice or eggs, use an insecticide specifically designed to treat head lice which is available from your local pharmacy (1) _____ follow the instructions carefully. (2) _____ , if you do not wish to use a chemical treatment, you can use a mechanical method which involves liberally applying conditioner to the hair and scalp and combing through with a long-toothed metal lice comb. Head lice live in the hair and feed on the scalp; (3) _____ each section of hair must be combed through carefully. This method needs to be repeated 2 or 3 times to ensure full eradication (4) _____ the chemical treatment should only be done once. If you find live lice in your child's hair after using an insecticide, you will know that this method has not worked and (5) _____ you will need to repeat the process using a different chemical compound. If your child has a particularly severe or recurring infestation, please seek further medical assistance. (6) _____, an oral medication exists which is very effective at eradicating head lice, but is only available on prescription from a doctor. (7) _____, head lice cannot survive for very long on personal items (8) _____ hats, bedding, carpets or furniture, so there is no need for excessive cleaning of these items. (9) _____, it is a good idea to wash your child's pillowcase in hot water. (10) _____, it is important to note that most infestations of head lice are short-lived and can be managed at home.

0	A	Significantly	B	By the way	C	**First**		
1	A	in addition to	B	and	C	also		
2	A	Particularly	B	Finally	C	Alternatively		
3	A	therefore	B	after that	C	whereas		
4	A	by the way	B	whereas	C	unlike		
5	A	incidentally	B	however	C	unfortunately		
6	A	Fortunately	B	Especially	C	Including		
7	A	In other words	B	For example	C	Incidentally		
8	A	includes	B	such as	C	even so		
9	A	All the same	B	For instance	C	As well as		
10	A	In addition to	B	Alternatively	C	Above all		

SPEAKING PRACTICE 2: WHAT WOULD YOU SAY?

What would you say when giving a clear and organised response to people in the following situations?

1. a patient who needs support to manage their medications
2. a patient who does not understand why they need to mobilise soon after surgery
3. a teenage school student who needs help managing their stress levels
4. a carer who would like respite options for the person they care for
5. a patient who needs clarification of the steps involved in changing a colostomy bag
6. the parent of an immunocompromised child who needs advice on infection prevention and control strategies in the home

SPEAKING PRACTICE 3: ROLE PLAY

ROLE PLAY 1

Work in pairs as healthcare professional and patient. Read your role play card to familiarise yourself with the task. Take a few minutes to plan what you are going to say. You can make notes during the preparation time if you wish.

> **BOOSTER TIP**
>
> For this task, demonstrate that you able to structure clear and organised spoken text to communicate your ideas.

ROLE PLAY 1

ROLE A: HEALTHCARE PROFESSIONAL **SETTING: MATERNITY WARD**

You are visiting the room of a healthy, 2-day-old baby. The parent has mentioned that extended family members wish to visit the new baby. You have some concerns around infection prevention and control regarding these visitors.

TASK

- Enquire about the health of the new baby.
- Find out if the baby has had any visitors. Remind the parent to tell all visitors to wash their hands with soap and water or use the alcohol-based rub provided on arrival to the ward.
- When asked, tell the parent that unfortunately the baby's grandmother should not visit as she may have had an infectious disease and may still be infectious.
- Acknowledge that the baby's grandmother will be disappointed. Explain to the parent that newborn babies are vulnerable to infection because their immune systems are not yet mature. Emphasise that while this baby is healthy, other babies on the ward may not be in such good health.
- Explain that the baby's aunt is also an infection risk so she should wear a mask when visiting and perform hand hygiene. The parents also need to be vigilant about their baby's health and report to the nurse on duty if the baby seems unwell.
- Explain the importance of hand hygiene to the parent.
- Inform the parent how to keep surfaces clean of urine, faeces and vomit.
- Reassure the parent that these basic infection control measures will become second nature in time and will help to protect the health of their baby.

ROLE PLAY 1

ROLE B: PATIENT   SETTING: MATERNITY WARD

You are the parent of a healthy, 2-day-old baby. You are talking to the healthcare professional on duty about family members who wish to visit the new baby.

TASK

- When asked, say that your baby appears to be doing well.
- When asked, say that your baby has not had visitors yet.
- Inform the healthcare professional that the baby's grandmother wishes to visit. She was recently very unwell with flu-like symptoms.
- Mention that the baby's grandmother will be very disappointed.
- Inform the healthcare professional that the baby's aunt is arriving on an international flight today and would like to visit the baby tomorrow.
- Ask what signs to look for in a sick baby and how to keep your baby safe from infection.
- Comment that there seems to be a lot of cleaning with a new baby.

ROLE PLAY 2

Work in pairs as healthcare professional and patient. Read your role play card to familiarise yourself with the task. Take a few minutes to plan what you are going to say. You can make notes during the preparation time if you wish.

ROLE PLAY 2

ROLE A: HEALTHCARE PROFESSIONAL **SETTING: GENERAL PRACTICE CLINIC**

Your patient is very unwell with flu-like symptoms. You suspect a case of influenza (the flu). You are advising the patient on treatment and returning to work.

TASK

- Enquire about the patient's symptoms.

- Ask how long your patient has had these symptoms.

- Inform your patient that they most likely have a strain of influenza (the flu).

- Instruct your patient to isolate at home and have plenty of rest and fluids.

- Remind your patient to wear a mask and use respiratory hygiene/cough etiquette if they need to go out. (Cover mouth and nose with a tissue when coughing/sneezing. Dispose of the used tissue. If no tissue available, cough/sneeze into bent elbow. Wash hands after coughing/sneezing.)

- Inform your patient that you are going to prescribe an antiviral medication which must be taken as soon as possible. (Antiviral medications for influenza are most effective at reducing the severity and duration of flu symptoms when the first dose is taken within 48 hours of the onset of symptoms.)

- Remind your patient that even with the antiviral medication, they will not be able to return to work immediately. (Exclusion periods apply to healthcare workers with acute infections. Your patient must not go to work if any signs or symptoms of a potentially infectious disease are present to ensure residents and other staff are not put at risk.)

- Ask your patient if they have been vaccinated against influenza this year.

- Instruct your patient to return to the clinic in 4 days for follow-up to ensure they are no longer infectious and can safely return to work.

ROLE PLAY 2

ROLE B: PATIENT SETTING: GENERAL PRACTICE CLINIC

You are a cook in an aged-care facility. You have had flu-like symptoms for 2 days. You are discussing your condition with a healthcare professional. You would like to return to work as soon as possible.

TASK

- When asked, say that your symptoms include a fever, cough, sore throat and feeling achy.
- When asked, say you have felt unwell for 2 days and have stayed at home.
- When told that you probably have influenza (the flu), ask about treatment options.
- Ask what you should do if you need to leave your home.
- Say that you have heard that antiviral medication can be effective.
- Ask when you might be able to return to work. (You are a cook in an aged-care facility.)
- Agree to adhere to the exclusion period as you do not want to expose others to your virus.
- When asked, say that you had your annual flu vaccine 4 days ago.
- Agree to return for follow-up prior to returning to work.

UNIT 8 MEDICAL EMERGENCIES

STUDY FOCUS

Reading: Identifying main ideas, locating specific information and recognising attitude, opinion and pronoun references

Vocabulary: Exploring medical emergencies

Writing: Selecting and transforming case notes to write medical letters

Exploring the topic

In pairs or groups, discuss the following questions.

- What are some common life-threatening medical emergencies?
- What are some common non life-threatening medical emergencies?
- What experience have you had with medical emergencies?

STUDY BOOST 1: READING AND VOCABULARY

READING 1

Read Texts 1-6 and choose the most suitable answer A, B or C. Write your answers in the space provided. An example (0) has been done for you.

BOOSTER TIP

For this task, identify **key words** in the questions and texts which will help you to locate the information you need to answer each question.

0   The notice is giving information about

    A   which staff should administer amiodarone.

    B   how amiodarone should be administered.

    C   when to administer amiodarone.

Antiarrhythmic agents

Amiodarone

A central venous catheter is recommended, although this route may not be feasible in a clinical emergency. If only peripheral access is available, concentrations should not exceed 2mg/mL for a maximum of 24 hours before attaining a central line as phlebitis is a known side effect.

1 Hospital staff involved in a clinical handover from emergency services
　A　have sole responsibility for validating the completion of the handover.
　B　must use checking strategies to ensure their understanding of the handover information is accurate.
　C　must not question the information provided by the emergency services personnel.

> **Notes – Handover to receiving staff**
>
> High quality handovers are essential for patient safety.
>
> In an emergency situation, clinical decisions may be driven by the information provided during the handover from emergency services personnel to the receiving hospital staff.
>
> At a minimum, a clinical handover must convey the patient's current condition, emerging or new critical information and any clinical concerns held by the attending staff.
>
> Emergency transfers can be fast-paced and chaotic as multiple clinicians may be present depending on the immediate patient care requirements. Ideally, emergency services personnel should have uninterrupted access to the ED clinicians for the duration of the handover. It is vital for the ED clinicians to use this opportunity to clarify and confirm the handover information by asking direct questions of the emergency services personnel.
>
> If the information given during the handover is incomplete or not clearly understood by the receiving staff, patient safety could be compromised. Miscommunication during the handover could also lead to diagnostic delays.
>
> Both parties must agree and sign off when the handover has been finalised.

2 According to the clinical practice notes, irrigation
　A　should not be initiated if there are signs of an open globe injury.
　B　prevents blindness as the result of a chemical injury.
　C　should be commenced at the earliest opportunity for all types of ocular trauma.

> **Clinical Practice Notes - Emergency Medicine for Student Nurses: Ocular Trauma**
>
> 9　Ocular Trauma – Chemical Injury
>
> 9.1 Chemical (acid and alkali) burns can lead to permanent visual impairment and disfigurement. Immediate irrigation of a chemical injury is critical to ensuring the best possible outcome.
>
> You will observe and assist with:
> - taking a visual acuity (VA) measurement
> - assessing the eye for an open globe injury (irrigation is contraindicated in open globe injuries)
> - instilling local anaesthetic drops to the affected eye/eyes
> - checking the pH of both eyes
> - irrigating the affected eye using an IV giving set and an undine eye irrigation unit
> - performing an eyelid eversion and sweeping the conjunctival fornices for debris or foreign bodies
>
> NOTE: Use soap and water (NOT alcohol-based sanitiser) to disinfect hands prior to donning gloves. Alcohol-based sanitiser can cause further irritation if it passes into the eye.

3   The purpose of this email is to
    A   report on procedural problems.
    B   explain the rationale for a change to procedures.
    C   request staff to reflect on procedures.

Central Women and Children's Hospital

Email

TO: Midwifery Team

SUBJECT: Preparation for Team Meeting

We are continuously striving to improve our continuity of care model for transfer of information during Category 2 – emergency caesarean section. Please refresh your knowledge of the guidelines: Transfer of information during Category 2 emergency caesarean section. These have been included in this email for your convenience.

Guidelines

To ensure the most accurate transfer of information and provide continuity of care for the mother, current guidelines for emergency caesarean deliveries where the decision-to-delivery interval is 60 minutes state that the midwife who has been caring for the mother antenatally/intrapartum _must_:

- inform the mother of the clinical picture and decision for caesarean section.
- obtain verbal consent and record consent in the mother's medical record.
- update the mother about changes to the clinical situation and record these discussions in the medical record.
- accompany the mother to theatre.
- participate in clinical discussions with all other staff involved in the delivery.

Please consider these guidelines before the next team meeting. We would like to draw on your clinical experience for discussion of the current guidelines at the meeting.

---

4   The extract informs us that
    A   merperidine has certain advantages over morphine.
    B   metoclopramide cannot be administered with morphine.
    C   tramadol may be preferable for patients with a pain score of 5.

Drugs for non life-threatening emergencies in a general practice setting

---

Initial management of severe acute pain in adults

Parenteral opioids have a place in the treatment of severe acute pain in general practice although practitioners must consider and exclude drug-seeking behaviour before administering opioids.

Furthermore, practitioners should prioritise non-opioid analgesia for initial pain management. Severe pain (7-10) can be managed with IV morphine sulfate and can also be given IM or SC. IV morphine sulfate has a rapid onset of action and can be titrated gradually to the desired analgesic effect to achieve effective pain relief for the patient.

Morphine should be avoided in patients with a known allergy.

Morphine is contraindicated in patients with respiratory insufficiency and depression since morphine can further decrease respiratory control. An immediate injection of naloxone is required to reverse the effects of morphine if a diagnosis of respiratory depression is made.

> Adverse reactions may include nausea, vomiting, sedation. Concomitant use of an antiemetic such as metoclopramide may reduce nausea and vomiting.
>
> Morphine is preferred to merperidine due to lower toxicity and greater efficacy. Merperidine has a high potential for dependence.
>
> For moderate pain (4-6), consider tramadol via slow IV or IM.

5   The objective of this extract from Dr Bentley's presentation is to
    A   advise residents not to seek input from other healthcare professionals.
    B   highlight the value of collaboration among all critical care team members.
    C   suggest that all senior nurses have more skills than resident doctors.

Extract from Dr Bentley's presentation about interprofessional communication in critical care

Effective communication is the basic requirement for all positive interaction, including successful teamwork, with other healthcare professionals in the emergency healthcare team.

Resident doctors are often required to take a leadership role within the emergency team, even though others may have more experience. As a junior resident, I realised that I needed to develop better interprofessional communication skills and be open to learning from other more experienced team members. To be specific, although I knew that some of the senior nurses had been working in emergency far longer than I had, I seldom included them in team communication. After I began to involve them directly, for instance, by asking them whether they had any further information to share about the patient, a much more cooperative working relationship within the team was established.

6   This case study highlights that
    A   clinical suspicions of foreign body aspiration can be confirmed or excluded through careful questioning.
    B   only an ENT specialist can diagnose foreign body aspiration.
    C   a negative history of choking excludes a diagnosis of foreign body aspiration.

Case study – 3-year-old child with foreign body in trachea

Prompt recognition and early treatment is critical to avoid complications associated with a missed foreign body.

A well-looking 3-year-old female presented to emergency. There was no initial choking episode and no signs of coughing or obvious respiratory distress. Her father, a former nurse, noticed that she was less energetic than usual and performed auscultation at home. He detected stridor, which prompted the emergency department presentation. Neither parent suspected foreign body aspiration. Following radiography, the emergency department physician confirmed foreign body aspiration.

The case was referred to an ENT specialist for management.

A small piece of raw carrot was subsequently removed from the trachea under general anaesthesia.

A discussion with the parents following the procedure revealed that a plate of raw vegetables had been given to older children earlier in the day.

Comments: Foreign body inhalation is frequently unwitnessed and may be denied by carers. Careful history-taking may arouse suspicion of the presence of a foreign body. A high degree of suspicion of foreign body aspiration is required in all cases of abnormal respiration in children.

Write your answers here.

0	1	2	3	4	5	6
B						

VOCABULARY PRACTICE 1A: MATCHING MEANING

The words and phrases in Column A appear in Texts 1-6. Choose the most suitable word or phrase from Column B for each word or phrase in Column A. Write your answers in the space provided. An example (0) has been done for you.

COLUMN A	COLUMN B
0 **interaction**	A to make a huge effort to achieve a goal
1 arouse suspicion	B weakened, damaged
2 unwitnessed	C to provoke uncertainty, distrust
3 feasible	D **reciprocal communication**
4 emerging	E to keep something/someone out
5 disfigurement	F to wash out an injury or organ with water or medication
6 strive	G suggested, recommended that a drug or treatment should not be used
7 contraindicated	H blemish, imperfection, scar
8 compromised	I achievable, practicable
9 irrigate	J not observed
10 exclude	K starting to appear

Write your answers here.

0	1	2	3	4	5	6	7	8	9	10
D										

VOCABULARY PRACTICE 1B: SENTENCE COMPLETION

Match the beginning of sentences in Column A with the most suitable ending in Column B. Write your answers in the space provided. An example (0) has been done for you.

COLUMN A		COLUMN B	
0	A 24-year-old male builder presented to the emergency department with a nail protruding	A	to a momentary lapse in concentration by a nail gun user.
1	The injury sustained was accidental and self-inflicted, due	B	was found to be limited.
2	Visual inspection of the injury revealed	C	no bone involvement.
3	The range of movement of the left little finger was assessed and	D	the nail was removed with a simple extraction.
4	There was no apparent sensory deficit to	E	expected without complication.
5	X-ray results revealed	F	was restored.
6	A local anaesthetic was administered and	G	with a topical antimicrobial dressing.
7	Minimal debridement was required	H	through the distal phalanx of the left little finger.
8	The finger was thoroughly irrigated with normal saline and treated	I	the affected hand.
9	Full range of movement	J	penetration of the volar soft tissue of the affected finger.
10	A tetanus booster was	K	administered because of the nature of the wound.
11	The patient was discharged home with instructions	L	to leave the dressing intact for 3 days.
12	A full recovery was	M	to ensure the edges of the wound were clean.

Write your answers here.

0	1	2	3	4	5	6	7	8	9	10	11	12
H												

READING 2

Texts A-F relate to staff training experiences in ST-elevation myocardial infarction.

Read Texts A-F and answer Questions 1-15.

BOOSTER TIP

For this task, read the text carefully to identify the information required to answer each question. Read the details closely to ensure clear understanding of the text and questions.

Staff training experiences in ST-elevation myocardial infarction: Reducing door-to-balloon time in percutaneous coronary intervention

TEXT A

ST-elevation myocardial infarction (STEMI) is a life-threatening medical emergency **which** is caused by the complete blockage of a coronary artery. Re-opening the blocked artery as quickly as possible is vital to restore blood flow to the heart. Percutaneous coronary intervention (PCI) is a nonsurgical procedure that is used to unblock a clogged or narrowed artery and involves inserting a catheter via the wrist or groin and inflating a small balloon at the end of that catheter, which clears the blockage. The best outcomes for the patient are achieved when the recommended door-to-balloon time of ≤90 minutes is met. Continuing professional development is essential for all medical professionals involved with this emergency procedure.

TEXT B

As a radiologic technologist who works exclusively in the cardiac catheterisation laboratory, Ray Tran appreciates training opportunities that broaden **his** knowledge and skill base as these enable him to perform his job more efficiently.

Ray explains, 'I recall one training session which was modelled on an unstable STEMI patient in a rapidly changing situation. The entire process was rehearsed, from arrival at the hospital to completing the PCI. All staff involved in managing the patient, including emergency services personnel, were present for the duration of the session. The interventional cardiologist was our mock patient and **he** gave real-time feedback about how we could improve our performances and response times. The session was designed to expedite our processes which would facilitate faster passage of the patient into the catheterisation laboratory. All participants agreed that it was a very productive session which highlighted the integral collaboration required when working in a dynamic environment.'

TEXT C

'Running a cardiac catheterisation laboratory requires multidisciplinary coordination. Ensuring that there is always someone on site with the relevant expertise to initiate catheterisation laboratory activation is critical, especially for STEMI patients **who** often present outside of the usual operating hours when the interventional cardiologist and catheterisation laboratory team are not immediately available. The cross-training of emergency physicians like myself to be able to rapidly identify STEMI cases and activate and prepare the catheterisation laboratory is an important part of achieving the goal door-to-balloon time of ≤90 minutes at our facility.

The cross-training sessions involve a member of the catheterisation laboratory team spending time with emergency department staff reviewing cases and highlighting where clinical processes could be further streamlined.

The catheterisation laboratory manager has confidence in the demonstrated effectiveness of the training which enables emergency department physicians to diagnose and prepare the patient for the PCI.'

TEXT D

A key responsibilty of Ruth Petersen's job as a cardiac catheterisation laboratory nurse is to closely monitor the patient during the procedure. 'Serious complications of cardiac catheterisation which result in morbidity or mortality are rare, but, unfortunately, **they** are inevitable in this line of work,' says Ruth.

'The training I find the most valuable for this role involves team sessions which focus on preparation for potential intraprocedural complications. Team members are presented with a specific complication for discussion and evaluation. We explore our individual responses to the issue and discuss possible outcomes. The objective of this training is to help us anticipate and proactively manage potential challenges which will positively impact door-to-balloon times.'

TEXT E

'I value informal feedback as much as formal feedback, perhaps even more so,' says Brendan Souza, a cardiac catheterisation laboratory manager. 'Informal conversations with colleagues in the corridor can provide an unexpected source of inspiration for change or improvement of systems in the workplace. For example, I had a chance conversation recently with a colleague. **She** mentioned her make-up artist daughter's creative organisation and storage of cosmetics using coloured boxes. This resulted in our adoption of dedicated colour-coded STEMI medication boxes containing all necessary medications, now located in both the emergency department and the catheterisation laboratory. The duplicate boxes enable medications to be quickly identified and accessed by staff in either location. When every second counts, I appreciate every innovative idea suggested by the team to make our processes even more efficient.'

TEXT F

A year ago, cardiothoracic intensive care nurse Michelle West began transitioning into a new role with the cardiac catheterisation laboratory team. After having worked with cardiac patients for 6 years, Michelle was able to adapt to the new position more easily than other nurses new to the team who had no previous cardiac critical care unit experience.

Michelle says, 'I knew in advance that the highly skilled team required rigorous training to achieve the desired door-to-balloon time of ≤90 minutes to treat a STEMI patient with PCI, but I was not fully aware of how much practical, intensive training was needed.

The first training session that I attended involved timed rehearsals of the three separate stages of treating a STEMI patient.

1. hospital arrival ➜ initial ECG
2. STEMI confirmation ➜ transfer to cardiac catheterisation laboratory
3. arrival at cardiac catheterisation laboratory ➜ inflating balloon

We were evaluated on the times we recorded as well as how well **we** responded to the impact of unanticipated challenges including fully occupied lifts and mock patients interrupting us to ask questions.'

Questions 1-6

Decide in which text, A, B, C, D, E or F, you can find the information mentioned in Questions 1-6. You may refer to each text more than once. Write your answers in the space provided. An example (0) has been done for you.

BOOSTER TIP

For this task, read the text carefully to locate the **specific information** required for each question. Read the details closely to ensure clear understanding of the text and questions.

In which text can you find information about

0 <u>a nurse preparing for a new position?</u>
1 major adverse clinical outcomes?
2 looking to discover new and different ideas?
3 a healthcare professional acting as a critically ill patient?
4 the importance of clear arteries?
5 training staff to be able to fulfil different roles?
6 chatting casually with co-workers about family members?

Write your answers here.

0	1	2	3	4	5	6
F						

Questions 7-10

Answer Questions 7-10 with a word or short phrase from Texts A-F. Each answer may include words, numbers or both.

7 What is the optimum time between arrival at emergency and PCI for a patient suffering from STEMI?
_____

8 Which two body parts can be used to access the affected coronary artery during PCI?
_____

9 What original idea prompted the development of colour-coded medication STEMI medication boxes?
_____

10 How did Michelle West's training replicate an authentic STEMI emergency?
_____

Questions 11-15

For Questions 11-15 choose the best answer A, B or C according to the information given in Texts A-F.

11 Brendan Souza believes informal communication
   A is not as important as formal feedback.
   B plays an important role in fostering change in the workplace.
   C is not relevant to the workplace.

12 Ray Tran describes one particularly memorable training session which
   A practised only one stage of managing a STEMI patient.
   B attracted positive comments from a STEMI patient.
   C demonstrated the importance of teamwork in an emergency environment.

13 Michelle West was better-suited to her new role than other nurses because
   A she knew she could achieve the optimum door-to-balloon time without much training.
   B she was very successful at problem-solving activities.
   C she had relevant prior work experience.

14 The cardiac catheterisation laboratory manager is convinced that multidisciplinary coordination is the best strategy for
   A mentoring staff who are critical of the laboratory processes.
   B developing teams with the expertise to provide a comprehensive service at all times.
   C training emergency physicians to perform PCI procedures on STEMI patients.

15 Ruth Petersen finds the most useful aspect of her training involves
   A learning how to avert negative outcomes for STEMI patients.
   B reviewing complete patient case histories with colleagues.
   C realising that morbidity or mortality due to complications from PCI are common.

Write your answers here.

11	12	13	14	15

VOCABULARY PRACTICE 2A: MATCHING REFERENCE PRONOUNS

Read through Texts A-F again. Look at the underlined pronouns in bold in each text. Match each pronoun listed in Column A with the word or expression it refers to in Column B. Write your answers in the space provided. An example (Example from Text B) has been done for you.

READING TEXT	COLUMN A	COLUMN B	
Example from Text B	**his**	i	complications of cardiac catheterisation
A	which	ii	Michelle West and fellow trainees
B	he	iii	STEMI
C	who	iv	STEMI patients
D	they	v	the interventional cardiologist
E	She	vi	a colleague
F	we	**vii**	**Ray Tran**

Write your answers here.

Example from Text B	A	B	C	D	E	F
vii						

VOCABULARY PRACTICE 2B: WORD FORMS

Look carefully at the text relating to interventional radiology. Choose the most suitable option A, B or C to complete each sentence. Write your answers in the space provided. An example (0) has been done for you.

Emergency care teams are **(0) recommended** to include an interventional radiologist among their multi-skilled experts. Although all radiologists are able to demonstrate a basic level of skill in (1) _____ interventional procedures, an interventional radiologist completes many years of (2) _____ training in complex life-saving interventional radiology procedures to treat trauma and acute emergencies.

Interventional radiology is often referred to as 'pinhole surgery' as it (3) _____ minimally invasive procedures conducted with needles, catheters and wires with the assistance of ultrasound, computed tomography (CT), x-ray or magnetic resonance imaging (MRI) scanning to track their precise (4) _____ .

Widespread (5) _____ for interventional radiology procedures over open and laparoscopic (keyhole) surgery is easily understood as they are less invasive, present less risk and pain and fewer complications, all of which lead to faster (6) _____ time and a shorter stay in hospital.

An integral function of interventional radiology is to control or prevent abnormal bleeding in any part of the body, such as (7) _____ bleeding from traumatic injuries sustained in a traffic accident, gastrointestinal bleeding from an ulcer or postpartum haemorrhage (PPH).

PPH is a life-threatening emergency (8) _____ from serious complications of childbirth, such as a torn artery, placental bleeding or more (9) _____ from uterine atony. An interventional radiology procedure, uterine artery embolisation, may be used to treat PPH.

During this minimally invasive procedure, very small particles of (10) _____ material, such as Gelfoam which usually dissolves within a few months, are mixed with a contrast solution and inserted into the uterine artery to stop further blood flow to the area. This can be life-saving and significantly reduces the risk of an emergency hysterectomy.

0	A **recommended**	B recommend	C recommendation
1	A performs	B performing	C performance
2	A specialised	B specialise	C specialising
3	A involvement	B involving	C involves
4	A positioned	B positioning	C reposition
5	A preferences	B preferential	C preference
6	A recover	B recovers	C recovery
7	A abdomen	B abdominal	C abdomens
8	A resulting	B results	C result
9	A commons	B common	C commonly
10	A embolic	B embolise	C embolising

Write your answers here.

0	1	2	3	4	5	6	7	8	9	10
A										

READING 3: COMPLETE THE SENTENCE

Read the following text about stress factors for staff in emergency healthcare. Choose the best phrase (A-K) to complete each sentence 1-10. Write your answers in the space provided. An example (0) has been done for you.

> **BOOSTER TIP**
>
> For this task, look carefully at both the meaning and the structure of the text to ensure it is cohesive and grammatically accurate.

Emergency healthcare professionals work in a challenging, high-stress environment, which demands considerable physical **(0) and mental resilience**. There are three main sources of stress associated with the work of emergency healthcare professionals. (1) _____ to the intense pressure they are under to make fast and accurate decisions regarding patients (2) _____ .

Unscheduled 'walk-in' presentations of unwell people to emergency departments contribute (3) _____ and anxiety for emergency doctors and nurses. In these situations, when members of the emergency team are meeting the patients for the first time, they do not have a complete (4) _____ or a letter of referral, which would help to inform their decisions.

The second potential stressor for those who work in emergency relates to unacceptable conduct of patients or visitors to emergency departments. In particular, emergency doctors and nurses are

(5) _____ or physically abused during episodes of violent behaviour by patients or visitors, especially those who are drug- or alcohol-affected. Responding to the needs of anxious family members requires immense empathy, energy and effective listening skills by the emergency team, (6) _____ manage while simultaneously balancing the demands of providing the best patient care.

The third important stressor that affects emergency doctors and nurses is the emotional impact of shocking injuries they encounter in the workplace, for example, (7) _____ a high-speed motorcycle accident, the serious burns to the face and body of a young child or a person with head trauma.

It is crucial that emergency doctors and nurses are aware of the warning signs of elevated adrenaline levels caused by long-term exposure to stress, such (8) _____ impatience, extreme fatigue and the increased risk of the more serious health issues of heart attack or stroke. They are recommended to protect their physical and mental health by (9) _____ into their daily routine outside of the workplace, including maintaining regular uninterrupted sleep patterns, participating in physical activities preferably outdoors and enjoying social interaction with friends and family.

Within the workplace, systematic exposure to significant trauma in emergency departments is widely acknowledged as being very difficult to overcome without support. (10) _____ an informal chat with a colleague, a general debrief session with team members to discuss a critical incident that has occurred or formal counselling arranged by a supervisor. All emergency doctors and nurses are strongly encouraged to access professional counselling services as a priority whenever they need to focus on their personal wellbeing.

A   those sustained by a person in

B   which can be very stressful to

C   **and mental resilience**

D   who need immediate medical attention

E   at risk of being mentally

F   This can be

G   as headaches, insomnia,

H   to a heightened sense of urgency

I   incorporating simple strategies

J   The first of these relates

K   medical history

Write your answers here.

0	1	2	3	4	5	6	7	8	9	10
C										

Discussion

1 What are the professional benefits of working in an emergency department?
2 How can emergency healthcare professionals ensure their ongoing physical and mental wellbeing?
3 What aspect of emergency care do you find the most interesting?

STUDY BOOST 2: WRITING

Selecting and transforming relevant case notes to write a medical letter

1 Selecting relevant case notes

The task and the case notes provide all the information you need to write a medical letter.

The purpose of the letter specified in the task determines which case notes you will need to select.

DO:

✔ Read the task carefully.

✔ Identify who you are writing to.

✔ Understand the purpose of the letter.

✔ Read the case notes carefully.

✔ Select the relevant case notes based on what the reader needs to know.

DO NOT:

✘ Include information that is not relevant to the purpose of the letter.

✘ Include information which is not presented in the case notes.

WRITING PRACTICE 1: SELECTING RELEVANT CASE NOTES

Read the task and the case notes and answer Questions 1-3.

You are a healthcare professional working at Cannonvale Hospital. Your patient is now ready to be discharged from hospital and transferred to a rehabilitation facility.

> **TASK**
>
> - Read the case notes and use the information given to write a Letter of Transfer for your patient Mr James Adams.
>
> - Your name is Dr Jacqueline Stratton.
>
> - You are writing to Dr Pamela Smith at Total Rehabilitation Centre, 76 West Avenue, Springfield.
>
> - In your letter, transform the relevant case notes into complete sentences. DO NOT USE NOTE FORM. Use a letter format.
>
> - Assume that today's date is 20 May 2021.

CASE NOTES
CANNONVALE HOSPITAL
PATIENT DETAILS

NAME:	James Adams
DOB:	4 April 1977 (44 years old)
NEXT OF KIN:	Michael Adams (brother)
ADMISSION DATE:	16 May 2021
DISCHARGE DATE:	20 May 2021
REASON FOR ADMISSION:	? CVA
DIAGNOSIS:	CVA caused by possible vasospasm
SOCIAL BACKGROUND:	Lives alone Works full time – personal trainer Former smoker (ceased at 20 y.o.) Minimal alcohol
FAMILY HISTORY:	Mother – angina Father – deceased MI aged 52 years
MEDICAL HISTORY:	Nil significant
MEDICATIONS:	None recorded
ALLERGIES:	None known
PRESENTATION AND ASSESSMENT:	Admitted via ambulance with right sided weakness esp. hand, slurred speech Sharp head pain LOC (loss of consciousness) approx. 30 secs Slightly confused (resolved), no complaints of pain BP 165/110 (high) Pulse 120 bpm (high) Temperature 37°C (normal) O² therapy given Admit for obs
MRI/CT head:	Unremarkable
TREATMENT AND MANAGEMENT:	Assisted ++ with ADLs Aspirin 81mg daily Physiotherapy – daily – restore hand function and regain balance ➜ slow improvement ➜ to rehab, 5-day program and reassess Speech therapy – daily – restore speech – good progress Monitored 4 days – BP 130/65 on discharge Pulse 80 bpm on discharge Mobile with supervision
DISCHARGE PLAN:	Discharge ➜ rehabilitation centre – hand function and balance Writing practice ++ Aspirin 81mg daily, review on discharge from rehab Discussion – Pt keen to return to full function for work

Questions 1-3

1 Who are you writing to?
_____

2 What is the purpose of the letter?
_____

3 Decide which case notes are relevant and should be included in the letter AND which case notes are <u>not</u> relevant and should not be included in the letter.

RELEVANT – INCLUDE	NOT RELEVANT – DO NOT INCLUDE
Patient's name – James Adams	Patient's next of kin – Michael Adams

2 Transforming case notes into complete sentences

Case notes are usually short and precise. Transforming relevant case notes into complete sentences requires the correct use of appropriate grammatical features. You must also ensure that the meaning of the sentences you write accurately conveys the information given in the case notes.

Read the examples below and notice how the grammatical features are used to help create complete sentences.

Articles	
EXAMPLE CASE NOTES	**EXAMPLE COMPLETE SENTENCES**
Pt - Mr Casey Gut symptoms 1-2 years - ? trigger	*I have not been able to identify **a** trigger for Mr Casey's ongoing gut symptoms of 1-2 years' duration.*
Pathology received 11/11/21 - LRTI	*Pathology results received on 11/11/21 indicate **a** lower respiratory tract infection.*
Pt – Mrs Lawson 1/9 - Discussed with family – transfer to palliative care ward 3 Sep.	*Following **a** discussion with her family, Mrs Lawson will be transferred to **the** palliative care ward on 3 September.*
ECG – severe primary hypothyroidism	***An** electrocardiogram indicated severe primary hypothyroidism.*

Auxiliary verbs	
EXAMPLE CASE NOTES	**EXAMPLE COMPLETE SENTENCES**
Pt – Mr Zhang Confined to bed – 3 days/toileting at bedside	*Mr Zhang **has** not ambulated from bed for 3 days and **has been** toileting at the bedside.*
Pt – Mrs Jackson Resume normal diet today – 1615	*Mrs Jackson **may** recommence drinking fluids and eating foods at 1615 today.*
Pt – Mr Young Medications: 4/12 - amitriptyline 5mg nocte (insomnia) review after 4 weeks	*I **will be** trialling Mr Young on amitriptyline (5mg at night) for insomnia.*
Pt – Mr White 14/2/2014 – DVT confirmed	*Mr White **was** diagnosed with deep vein thrombosis on 14/2/2014.*

Conjunctions

EXAMPLE CASE NOTES	EXAMPLE COMPLETE SENTENCES
Pt – Mrs McIntyre Discussion with Pt – Pt complains of pain, Pt not taking pain relief as directed	Mrs McIntyre reports uncontrolled arthritis pain, **but** it should be noted that she is not compliant with the pain relief management plan I have previously recommended.
Allergies - none known	There are no known food, drug **or** environmental allergies.
Pt – Miss Armstrong Sudden onset – admit for obs overnight	Miss Armstrong remained in hospital for observation overnight **due to** the sudden onset of symptoms.
Pt – Ms Spencer Discussion with Pt – Pt requested referral to lactation consultant – Pt to continue breastfeeding and returning to work p/t	Ms Spencer requested a referral to a lactation consultant for advice **because** she intends to continue to breastfeed **when** she returns to work part-time.

Prepositions

EXAMPLE CASE NOTES	EXAMPLE COMPLETE SENTENCES
Pt – Olivia Harrison Reason for ED presentation – acute onset shortness of breath	Olivia Harrison presented **to** the emergency department **with** acute onset shortness **of** breath.
Nappy rash – apply zinc oxide when changing nappy	A zinc oxide cream should be applied **to** the affected area **at** every nappy change **to** relieve the symptoms **of** nappy rash.
MRI - Ventricles and basal cisterns – normal limits	The ventricles and basal cisterns appear **within** normal limits.
Pt – Mrs Halcrow Discussion with Pt re: care following laparoscopy – no heavy lifting, 10kgs max for 4 weeks	Mrs Halcrow has been advised not to lift more **than** 10 kilograms **for** 4 weeks **after** laparoscopic surgery.

Pronouns

EXAMPLE CASE NOTES	EXAMPLE COMPLETE SENTENCES
Dressings – leave for 5 days, check for wound discharge, if clear remove dressing and air	The wound dressings are to remain in place. After 5 days, remove the dressings and if there is no discharge from the wounds, leave **them** open to the air.
Pt – Mr Rovira Medications: paroxetine (20mg/day) – do not cease taking suddenly	Mr Rovira takes paroxetine (20mg/day). **This** medication should not be discontinued suddenly.
Discussed with mother – how to monitor baby's O^2 supply when home	Our discussion included how to monitor **her** baby's oxygen supply at home.

Relative pronouns

EXAMPLE CASE NOTES	EXAMPLE COMPLETE SENTENCES
Pt – Ms Fisher 1 Nov – hard bump to eye socket, saw stars, Pt reports changes to vision 30 Nov – Pt complaining of changes to vision	Ms Fisher is experiencing problems with her eyes **which** she first noticed after a minor head injury a month ago.
Pt – Mr Marshall Plan: refer to haematologist to investigate unusual blood test results - ? lymphopenia	Thank you for seeing Mr Marshall, **whom** I consulted today regarding unexplained lymphopenia.
Pt – Mr Mitchell Current BMI 38.3 Discussion – Pt requests dietician support to ↓ weight	Mr Mitchell, **whose** current BMI is 38.3, wishes to discuss weight loss options with you.
Pt – Mr Martinez Medications: enoxaparin (S/C – Pt to administer daily) - SVT left leg, regressing	Mr Martinez has been self-administering enoxaparin by subcutaneous injection for extensive SVT left leg, **which** has been regressing.

WRITING PRACTICE 2: COMPLETE THE SENTENCE

Read the case notes and then read the Letter of Discharge for patient Anja Cameron. Choose the most suitable word from the box to complete each sentence. There is one extra word which you do not need to use. Write your answers in the space provided. An example (0) has been done for you.

CASE NOTES
BELLEVUE CHILDREN'S HOSPITAL
PATIENT DETAILS

NAME:	Anja Cameron, 8 years old
DOB:	30/08/2013
NEXT OF KIN:	Zoe Cameron (mother)
ADMISSION DATE:	16/12/2021 2017
DISCHARGE DATE:	17/12/2021 0808
REASON FOR ADMISSION:	Pain to left neck
DIAGNOSIS:	Spasmodic torticollis
ASSESSMENT:	Pain score 10/10 – left neck
	Pt crying, screaming
	Cannot move neck - ? cause
	TPR – normal
	BP – normal
	Recently well
TREATMENT AND MANAGEMENT:	Observe overnight
	Fentanyl (IN) – loading dose 1.5mcg/kg, repeat 30 mins – monitor for respiratory depression, hypotension, nausea, vomiting
	Paracetamol – 7mL by mouth
	Pt vomited – 0320
DISCHARGE PLAN:	Cease all pain relief
	↑↑ freedom of movement
	Rest 24-48 hrs
	Re-present asap if symptoms appear

LETTER OF DISCHARGE

| has had | due to | her | at | **the** | which | were |
| and | she | therefore | a | has been | however | on |

Anja Cameron, aged 8, presented to **(0) the** emergency department at Bellevue Children's Hospital (1) _____ 16 December 2021. She was in a high level of distress and experiencing (2) _____ significant amount of pain to the left neck. She was kept overnight for observation (3) _____ the sudden onset of pain without obvious cause. She (4) _____ no recent signs of illness or infection.

On examination, her vital signs were stable (5) _____ there were no symptoms other than a high level of neck pain and the inability to move (6) _____ head.

The diagnosis was spasmodic torticollis.

Intranasal fentanyl and oral paracetamol (7) _____ administered to relieve the pain. Anja was monitored overnight. She vomited once (8) _____ 0320.

On discharge, Anja was not exhibiting additional symptoms and (9) _____ was moving much more freely. She is no longer in need of pain relief, (10) _____ is reassuring.

She (11) _____ advised to rest for 24-48 hours, (12) _____, should urgently re-present should additional symptoms appear.

Write your answers here.

0	the
1	
2	
3	
4	
5	
6	
7	
8	
9	
10	
11	
12	

WRITING PRACTICE 3: COMPLETE THE SENTENCE

Read the case notes and then read the Letter of Referral for patient Mrs Emma Casella. Complete each sentence with the most suitable word or phrase. You will need to ensure that your answers match the information given in the case notes and are grammatically correct. Write your answers in the space provided. Two examples, (00) and (0), have been done for you.

CASE NOTES
GENERAL PRACTICE CLINIC
PATIENT DETAILS

NAME:	Emma Casella
DOB:	29 September 1962 (59 years old)
NEXT OF KIN:	Stewart Ashcroft (partner)
SOCIAL BACKGROUND:	Divorced; lives with partner 3 adult children Works full time – solicitor
FAMILY HISTORY:	Mother – frequent memory loss Maternal grandmother – bowel cancer age 60s
MEDICAL HISTORY:	Osteoporosis – crush fracture at T5 COPD (ex-smoker) 30 Jun 2020 - Pt reports intermittent indigestion over past 2 years 1 Dec 2021 – ED presentation – epigastric/chest pain and vomiting, ECG – normal, not cardiac
SURGICAL HISTORY:	Appendicectomy - child Nov 2012 - BCC R upper lip
MEDICATIONS:	12% salicylic acid in aqueous cream – apply daily to forearms Ca 600mg tablets - 1 at night Vitamin D capsules 25mcg (equiv. vit D3 1000 IU) – 2 daily Fluticasone propionate/salmeterol xinafoate MDI (250/25) 120 dose – 2 puffs twice daily
ALLERGIES:	Shellfish
PRESENTING COMPLAINT:	3 Dec 2021: 3 episodes substernal pain, vomiting, lasting +/- 10 hrs Onset 4 days ago Occurs after evening meal Pt took OTC antacid – little improvement; appetite ↓ O/E – no RUQ tenderness ? Biliary colic ? cause
PATHOLOGY RESULTS:	Received 3 Dec 2021 - LFTs mild elevation
PLAN:	Request pathology – FBC, ESR, LFTs – Pt to do today Request USS – upper abdomen – this week ? GOR – trial PPI (proton pump inhibitor) for 2 weeks Codeine/paracetamol 2 tabs when necessary Referral to hepatic and biliary surgeon for advice and management

LETTER OF REFERRAL

Thank you for seeing Mrs Emma Casella (59 years old), **(00) whom** I consulted today, for assessment and management of suspected **(0) biliary colic**. Mrs Casella has a history of (1) _____ of approximately two years' duration and is experiencing increasing episodes of substernal pain with (2) _____, with each episode lasting approximately (3) _____. She took an (4) _____ antacid on each occasion. However, she reports that this was of minimal assistance. Her (5) _____ is diminished.

No (6) _____ tenderness was experienced at any time during examination.

Liver function tests (3/12/21) indicate mild elevation.

Mrs Casella (7) _____ the emergency department at Westside Hospital on 1/12/21 where she was checked for cardiac involvement, (8) _____ was subsequently excluded.

I prescribed (9) _____ to be taken when necessary to manage severe pain. I will (10) _____ Mrs Casella on a proton pump inhibitor prior to her seeing you to determine whether (11) _____ is the cause of these symptoms.

I have requested an ultrasound scan (upper abdomen), the results of which I will forward to you when (12) _____ become available.

If you require further information, please do not hesitate to contact me.

Yours sincerely

Dr Randall Thomas

Write your answers here.

00	whom
0	biliary colic
1	
2	
3	
4	
5	
6	
7	
8	
9	
10	
11	
12	

WRITING PRACTICE 4: SELECTING AND TRANSFORMING CASE NOTES

Read the case notes and then read the Letter of Discharge for patient Mr Edward Gomez to the patient's general practitioner, Dr Krupa. Choose the most suitable phrase (A-T) to complete each sentence 1-15. There are 4 extra phrases which you do NOT need to use. Write your answers in the space provided. An example (0) has been done for you.

CASE NOTES
GREEN VALLEY HOSPITAL
PATIENT DETAILS

NAME:	Edward Gomez
DOB:	13 November 1950 (71 years old)
NEXT OF KIN:	Helen Gomez (wife)
SEEN IN ED:	1 November 2021 (0900 – 2130)
REASON FOR PRESENTATION:	LOC (loss of consciousness) – approx. 2 mins – collapsed at home
SOCIAL BACKGROUND:	Retired
	Lives with wife
FAMILY HISTORY:	Mother – died of bowel cancer
	Father – late onset IDDM, renal failure
MEDICAL HISTORY:	Hypertension (ongoing management)
MEDICATIONS:	Methyldopa (250mg daily)
ALLERGIES:	None known
PRESENTATION AND ASSESSMENT:	Laceration – left ear, 1cm deep
	No infective symptoms
	No stroke symptoms
	Normal neurological examination
	Normal cardiorespiratory examination
	Symptoms resolved within 12 hours
CT head/angio:	No intra cerebral haemorrhage
	No evidence of large established cerebral infarction
	Chronic white matter ischaemic changes
	Scattered atherosclerosis of the large arteries of the neck without evidence of a high-grade focal stenosis
	No evidence of carotid or vertebral artery dissection
	Normal CT angiogram of the brain with no evidence of a large vessel occlusion

DIAGNOSIS:	Most likely transient global amnesia
	? TIA
TREATMENT AND MANAGEMENT:	Left ear sutured
	12 hours observation
	TPR – normal
	ECG – normal sinus rhythm
	Aspirin – 50mg given
DISCHARGE PLAN:	Discharge home
	Wife to organise outpatient echocardiogram, Holter monitoring and MRI brain
	Wife to remove dressing to ear in 3 days; sutures will dissolve
	Increase aspirin to daily 100mg
	GP to monitor BP and uptitrate anti-HTN as required
	Follow up at hospital outpatient clinic in 2 weeks - appointment made 15/11/21

Dear Dr Krupa

Re: Mr Edward Gomez (aged 71)

Mr Gomez presented to the emergency department at Green Valley Hospital **(0) after collapsing at home.** He lost consciousness (1) _____ and suffered a 1cm deep laceration (2) _____.

He displayed no infective symptoms and (3) _____ of stroke. His neurological and cardiorespiratory examinations (4) _____.

A CT head/angiogram (5) _____. Of note were chronic ischaemic changes to white matter. The most probable diagnosis is transient global amnesia, however, TIA (6) _____.

Mr Gomez's ear was sutured (7) _____ a waterproof dressing. He (8) _____ for 12 hours and his vital signs were normal. No (9) _____ in ECG. Aspirin (50mg) was administered. The symptoms resolved (10) _____.

Mr Gomez was discharged home (11) _____, Helen, who will organise outpatient appointments on his behalf for echocardiogram, Holter monitoring and MRI – brain. He (12) _____ his daily dose of aspirin to 100mg.

Helen will remove (13) _____ the ear after 3 days.

Please continue to monitor Mr Gomez's blood pressure (14) _____ medications.

A (15) _____ has been made at the Green Valley Hospital Outpatient Clinic on 15/11/21.

Please do not hesitate to contact me if you require further information.

Yours sincerely,

Dr Bernard Small

A within 12 hours
B were both normal
C **after collapsing at home**
D and dressed with
E definitive diagnosis
F was observed
G is to increase
H for approximately 2 minutes
I normal sinus rhythm
J in the care of his wife
K the dressing to
L there was no indication
M follow-up appointment
N abnormality was detected
O was oriented to his surroundings
P was largely unremarkable
Q for review of hypertension
R is also a possibility
S to his left ear
T to commence hypertension

0	after collapsing at home
1	
2	
3	
4	
5	
6	
7	
8	
9	
10	
11	
12	
13	
14	
15	

WRITING EXTENSION TASK

Read the task and the case notes in Writing Practice 1 and use the information given to write a Letter of Transfer. Write your letter in the space provided. A sample answer is provided in the Answer Key.

Write your letter here.

UNIT 9 — FOCUS ON COMMON ERRORS 2: FORMAL AND INFORMAL LANGUAGE

STUDY FOCUS

Writing and Speaking: Developing awareness of using formal and informal language appropriately to achieve clear communication in a range of healthcare settings.

Exploring the topic

In pairs or groups, discuss the following questions.

- Why is it important to know when to use formal or informal language in healthcare settings?
- What are some healthcare scenarios where you would use formal words and expressions?
- What are some healthcare scenarios where you would use informal words and expressions?

STUDY BOOST 1

Using formal words and expressions in healthcare settings

Formal communication using standard English in healthcare settings enhances comprehensibility for all audiences. It is important to use formal language when:

- writing documents, including letters of referral or letters of discharge, staff handbooks, patient and carer information leaflets and professional emails.
- conducting healthcare staff induction and training.
- providing information and giving instructions to patients and families.

Characteristic elements of formal language reflect:

- **standard language:** official; polite, grammatically accurate style of writing and speaking.

    NOTE: Idioms are **not** appropriate in formal communication.

    Are you **back on your feet** after your illness? ✗

    Have you **recovered** from your illness? ✓

- **discipline-specific jargon** used appropriately between medical professionals, for example, NKDA (no known drug allergy), sutures (stitches), idiopathic (referring to a disease or condition of uncertain origin).

    NOTE: Jargon is **not** usually appropriate when communicating with patients and other non-medically-trained people as it may cause doubt or confusion.

- **an impersonal perspective**, which rarely uses personal pronouns – I, we or you. Passive verb structures are often used, for example: A coronary angiogram **was scheduled** for the patient.

- **full word forms**, for example: do not ✓ don't ✗; is not ✓ isn't ✗

- **longer and more complex sentences.**

Task 1

Matching formal with informal language

Match each example of formal language in Column A with the most suitable expression of informal language from Column B. Write your answers in the space provided. An example (0) has been done for you.

> **BOOSTER TIP**
> - Look carefully at the language features in the formal and informal sentences. Think about each situation to understand how context helps with choosing the most suitable language style in spoken and written communication.

	COLUMN A: FORMAL LANGUAGE		COLUMN B: INFORMAL LANGUAGE
0	<u>I would like to apologise for the delay to the start of the meeting.</u>	A	This report's about comparing the results of the two most recent blood tests.
1	All treatment options **are being considered** by the patient.	B	After the patient was admitted to the ICU, she started a treatment of broad-spectrum antibiotics.
2	The medical student **is scheduled to observe** an inguinal hernia repair today.	C	We need to do more histological staining to check out the immune-architecture of the removed lymph node.
3	Following admission to the intensive care unit, the patient **was initiated on** a treatment of broad-spectrum antibiotics.	D	The patient is thinking about all treatment options.
4	A structural abnormality in the brain **was indicated** in the computed tomography (CT) scans.	E	The medical student is timetabled to watch an inguinal hernia repair today.
5	Further histological staining **is required** to assess the immune-architecture of the excised lymph node.	F	<u>I'm sorry for the late start to the meeting.</u>
6	This report **concerns** a comparative analysis of the two most recent blood test results.	G	The CT scans showed up a structural abnormality in the brain.

Write your answers here.

0	1	2	3	4	5	6
F						

STUDY BOOST 2

Using informal expressions in healthcare settings

Informal language is more personal than formal language. It is frequently used by staff in healthcare settings to establish and maintain a relationship of confidence and trust when communicating:

- with colleagues in casual conversation.
- with patients about their interests, families and daily activities.
- with families and caregivers.

Distinctive features of informal language include:

- **phrasal verbs:** A phrasal verb combines a verb with a preposition to create a new meaning, for example, 'to pass out' means 'to faint, become unconscious'.
- **personal pronouns** - I, we, you.
- **contracted word forms,** for example: it's ✔ (it is) ; hasn't ✔ (has not) ; I'm ✔ (I am).
- **shorter and simpler sentences.**

Task 2

Matching informal phrasal verbs with formal English meaning

Match each example of informal phrasal verbs in Column A with the most suitable meaning in Column B. Write your answers in the space provided. An example (0) has been done for you.

BOOSTER TIP
• Look carefully at the common phrasal verbs in the informal sentence examples. Try to understand the meaning of the phrasal verb in each sentence from the context.
• Think about how you might use these phrasal verbs in your own communication. What would help you to decide when to use a phrasal verb and when to use a standard English expression?

	COLUMN A: PHRASAL VERB + SENTENCE EXAMPLE	COLUMN B: MEANING OF PHRASAL VERB
0	**pass out** **The patient passed out when he stood up after his dental treatment.**	A swell
1	come around I have no idea how long it took me to **come around** after I fainted.	B reschedule to an earlier time
2	put up with I don't think I can **put up with** this pain any longer. It's very bad.	C die
3	throw up Could I have a basin please? I am going to **throw up**.	D determine

UNIT 9 FOCUS ON COMMON ERRORS 2: FORMAL AND INFORMAL LANGUAGE

4	come down with You said it's been two days since you **came down with** these symptoms? Is that right?	E	persist, stay, linger longer than expected
5	go down Please give this medication to the child every 4 hours until her temperature **goes down.**	F	survive a serious illness or operation
6	get over How long does it usually take to **get over** food poisoning?	G	stop doing something that has become a habit
7	break out (in spots) Teenagers often feel self-conscious when they **break out** in spots.	H	investigate
8	put off It's against medical advice to **put off** the surgery any longer.	I	become infected with/contract an infectious disease
9	pass away Mrs Hawkins **passed away** at the age of 86.	J	tolerate, endure an unpleasant situation
10	fight off What do you use to **fight off** a sore throat or a cold?	K	give/take a measured amount of medication
11	puff up During pregnancy, you should elevate your legs frequently to stop your feet and ankles from **puffing up**.	L	<u>**faint/lose consciousness**</u>
12	pull through Luckily, our dog **pulled through** the emergency surgery after being hit by a car.	M	discontinue, stop taking medication
13	take up i) Mr Beker **took up** a new exercise regime to improve his cardiac health. ii) The amount of glucose **taken up** by abnormal tissues is measured by PET/CT.	N	eliminate
14	cut out **Cutting out** excess salt in your diet is strongly recommended.	O	gradually weaken and disappear (e.g. symptoms, side effects)
15	give up Global health campaigns encourage **giving up** smoking.	P	regurgitate, often describes vomiting in animals

COLUMN A: PHRASAL VERB + SENTENCE EXAMPLE	COLUMN B: MEANING OF PHRASAL VERB
16 flare up Although her chronic pain was mostly well-controlled by medication, it did **flare up** occasionally.	Q become lower/reduce
17 stick around My cough is still **sticking around** even though my cold has gone.	R postpone
18 pick up Some patients prefer telehealth consultations as they worry they will **pick up** a bug from other patients if they have to sit in a doctor's waiting room.	S regain consciousness
19 figure out The medical team have noted her symptoms, but they have not yet **figured out** a diagnosis.	T recover (from)
20 come off I feel really well now. How soon can I **come off** this medication?	U i) adopt/start something new ii) absorb
21 bring forward My appointment was **brought forward** from 10am to 9am because the doctor had to attend a meeting at 10am.	V resist, overpower
22 wear off The patient will be monitored in recovery until the effects of the anaesthetic **wear off**.	W suddenly appear (e.g. skin irritation, acne)
23 bring something up Cats can often be seen retching before **bringing up** a hairball.	X show signs of an illness that is not very serious (e.g. a cold)
24 look into We need to **look into** the underlying cause of this rash.	Y spontaneously occur from time to time (e.g. symptoms of an ongoing chronic medical condition)
25 dose up on Is there anything I can **dose up on** to prevent motion sickness?	Z vomit (i.e. forceful ejection of stomach contents)

Write your answers here.

0	1	2	3	4	5	6	7	8	9	10	11	12
L												

13	14	15	16	17	18	19	20	21	22	23	24	25

WRITING PRACTICE: SENTENCE TRANSFORMATION

Part 1

For Questions 1-5, transform the sentences using informal language into sentences using formal language. Complete the second sentence so that it has a similar meaning to the first sentence, using the word given in bold. Do not change the word given. Use between 2 and 5 words including the word given. An example (00) has been done for you.

00 required

The patient needs to be able to mobilise independently before leaving hospital.

The patient **is required to** be mobilising independently prior to discharge.

1 postponed

The hospital is going to put off all non-essential elective surgery for the next two weeks.

All non-essential elective surgery _____ for the next two weeks.

2 infected

If children do not wash their hands thoroughly when they are in a childcare setting, they are at risk of picking up an illness, such as gastroenteritis.

Thorough hand washing can minimise the risk of children in childcare settings _____ an illness, such as gastroenteritis.

3 investigating

The latest advances in diabetes monitoring systems are being looked into by technology experts.

Technology experts _____ the latest advances in diabetes monitoring systems.

4 absorbed

Regular phlebotomy treatment is used to reduce excess iron which is taken up by the liver in haemochromatosis sufferers.

Treatment to reduce excess iron _____ the liver in haemochromatosis sufferers includes regular phlebotomy.

5 rescheduled

The surgery was brought forward because the patient's condition was deteriorating rapidly.

The surgery _____ earlier time because the patient's condition was deteriorating rapidly.

Part 2

For Questions 6-10, transform the sentences using formal language into sentences using informal language. Complete the second sentence so that it has a similar meaning to the first sentence, using the word given in bold. Do not change the word given. Use between 2 and 5 words including the word given. An example (0) has been done for you.

0   about
Instructions in this leaflet concern post-cataract surgery eyecare.
This leaflet **is about how** to care for the eye after having cataract surgery.

6   get
Recovery after a tonsillectomy usually takes up to two weeks.
It usually takes up to two _____ tonsillectomy.

7   flared
Daisuke described the heightened anxiety he always experienced whenever his eczema symptoms suddenly recurred.
Daisuke talked about the increased anxiety he always felt whenever his eczema symptoms _____ unexpectedly.

8   puffed
After consuming strawberries, Sophie developed a rash on her face, her lips became swollen and she began vomiting.
Sophie started vomiting, her lips _____ and a rash appeared on her face after eating strawberries.

9   put
Russell had tried many unsuccessful home remedies to resolve a fungal nail infection before admitting he could no longer endure the pain and arranged a consultation with a podiatrist.
After trying many unsuccessful fungal nail home remedies, Russell made an appointment with a podiatrist because he _____ the pain any longer.

10   throwing
Serious side effects of cancer therapy treatments include extreme fatigue, hair loss and uncontrolled vomiting.
Feeling extremely fatigued, losing your hair and _____ uncontrollably are all serious side effects of cancer therapy treatments.

SPEAKING PRACTICE: MULTIPLE CHOICE

Read the context for each question and note who the speakers are. Choose the most appropriate response for each context. A is written in a formal style. B is written in an informal style. Write your answers in the space provided. An example (0) has been done for you.

0 Two aged care nurses, Julio and Su Jin, are chatting during their break time. Julio asks Su Jin to confirm their plans to meet up in their free time next weekend. Su Jin replies:

A I apologise but I have to cancel. The revised roster indicates that I have been scheduled to work.

B Sorry, no I can't make it. I'm rostered on here for an extra shift.

1 Radiographer Alex is positioning an elderly patient on the ultrasound table for a direct cortisone injection into the hip joint. Alex explains:

A For this procedure, you are required to remain immobile on the ultrasound table. The exact injection site will be located with the assistance of the scan probe. Please stay in the waiting room for 30 minutes following the procedure.

B Just hop up on the table and stretch out. I'll look and see where I have to put the needle in. When we are done, go and hang out in the waiting room for a while.

2 Nurse Jill Gibbons is introducing herself to patients in the ward at the start of her shift.

A Good morning. I am Nurse J Gibbons. I am responsible for your health status. Your clinical observations will be recorded regularly and your medications administered as per the instructions of the doctor.

B Hello. My name's Jill. I'll be looking after you today. I'm going to be seeing you quite a lot through the day when I take your observations and give you your medications. If you need my help, I'll be around, so just press your buzzer.

3 Lymphoma care nurse Donna is with patient Mrs Dean (56 years) who has been diagnosed recently with Hodgkin's lymphoma. Mrs Dean is feeling very anxious. Donna is responding to Mrs Dean's questions about treatment and some potential ongoing side effects.

A One dose of chemotherapy will be administered every 2-3 weeks for a period of 6 months. Depression and extreme fatigue can be experienced for up to six months following the last cycle of treatment. You are expected to attend post-treatment medical consultations.

B You'll most likely have chemotherapy every 2-3 weeks for 6 months. You may feel depressed and very tired for several months after finishing the treatment. Your doctor will set up ongoing appointments with you to check on how you are coping.

4 Dentist Dr Wan is providing induction training in his practice to new dental assistant Oliver about glove-wearing protocols in the treatment room.

   A New examination gloves are to be worn during all patient treatment. Hand hygiene protocols are to be completed before donning new gloves and again after doffing used gloves following the treatment of each patient.

   B Wash your hands and put on new gloves. Don't forget to wash your hands again after you take off and throw away the used gloves.

5 Nurse Chinayi is talking to an 8-year-old child, Han, who is suffering from asthma symptoms.

   A Good afternoon Han. Your airways are constricted, your breathing is laboured and coughing is present. Using a spacer with Ventolin is recommended to assist you.

   B Hello Han. How are you feeling? I can hear you are wheezing and you are still coughing a lot. Don't worry, I'll help you – here's your spacer and Ventolin.

6 Senior nurse Patrick is training a cohort of student nurses in how to record clinical patient notes.

   A There is a standard protocol to follow when writing a patient's clinical notes. Always verify the patient details, identify the focus of the note, record the date and time and sign off with your name and position title.

   B Let me tell you a few things about making notes about patients. First, check you have the right name for the patient, say what you have found out about the patient and write your name.

7 Nurse Mattia is talking to patient carer, John, whose wife, Emma (45 years old) is being discharged from hospital after knee replacement surgery.

   A Assistance will be required with showering and dressing. Mobilisation with crutches will continue. Pain relief is to be administered as per the doctor's instructions. Aspirin is to be taken daily for 6 weeks. The vacuum-assisted wound closure bandage is to be removed on Day 7.

   B Emma will need assistance with showering and dressing. She will continue to mobilise with her crutches. You will need to make sure that she takes her pain relief as per the doctor's instructions. She also needs to take aspirin every day for the next 6 weeks. Her pressure bandage should be taken off in one week's time. Written instructions are here in this discharge pack.

8   Hand therapist Seamus is talking to 12-year-old Jeong-hun, who dislocated his finger playing handball last week and is now presenting to the hand therapy clinic with his finger splinted and with an x-ray that was taken after the dislocation had been reduced.

   A   The x-ray indicates that the proximal interphalangeal joint was successfully reduced after dislocation. A customised thermoplastic splint to support the damaged ligaments and tendons will be created for you. Compliance with a prescribed regime of safe mobilisation exercises is essential to minimise swelling and develop increased range of motion in the finger.

   B   Let's take a look at your finger Jeong-hun. What I am going to do today is wrap your finger in a compression bandage. That will help to reduce the swelling. Then I am going to make a customised splint for you to stop your finger popping out again. Finally I am going to show you some special exercises to do at home that will strengthen your finger.

9   Consultant Dr Chiu is presenting to junior residents about the treatment plan of a patient diagnosed with a basal cell carcinoma to the superior helix (right auricle).

   A   A local anaesthetic will be administered. The basal cell carcinoma will be excised using Mohs surgery until the surrounding tissue is clear of cancer cells. Reconstruction will be undertaken with a full thickness skin graft.

   B   I will give a local anaesthetic to numb the outer ear and then cut out the tumour. If necessary, I will put a skin graft over the wound and stitch it on.

10 Emergency nurse Darlene is talking to patient Thiago, who has presented with an eye injury.

   A   There is a foreign body on the corneal surface. The doctor will examine your eye for signs of corneal abrasion and employ anaesthetic eye drops prior to removal of the foreign object.

   B   You have a small speck of dirt on the surface of your eye. The doctor will be here shortly to take it out for you and check that your eye hasn't been scratched.

Write your answers here.

0	1	2	3	4	5	6	7	8	9	10
B										

UNIT 10 — CONSOLIDATION 2 (UNITS 6-9)

READING PRACTICE

Read the following text about Parkinson's disease. For Questions 1-8, choose the most suitable answer A, B, C or D. Write your answers in the space provided.

Parkinson's disease

Apprehension and disbelief are common reactions for a person being given a preliminary diagnosis of suspected Parkinson's disease (PD). This person may question the reliability of the evaluation and seek alternative explanations for their symptoms. This is understandable, to some extent, as it is widely known that there is no specific objective medical test currently in use that can conclusively diagnose PD. A consultation with a neurologist specialising in PD is strongly recommended at the earliest opportunity for further investigation.

While emphasising that each person's experience of PD is unique, the neurologist is skilled at recognising common symptoms, including much slower physical movement known as bradykinesia, unusual gait, stooped posture, rigid facial muscles and hand tremor, which result from the degeneration of dopaminergic neurons in the area of the brain afflicted by PD and the consequent reduction of dopamine. Medication, such as a carbidopa-levodopa combination, which is converted into dopamine in the brain, is prescribed to ease body stiffness and is fundamental to PD treatment. Significant improvement in the patient's motor skills after taking the medication helps to confirm a suspected Parkinson's diagnosis.

Besides the serious disruption to gross motor skills, many sufferers of PD become aware that, as the disease progresses, conversation is increasingly challenging. Some patients may feel disorientated and may need to clarify and structure their thoughts before speaking. If patients are anxious that their language production is too slow to make a positive contribution to the conversation, they may start to speak, but then withdraw from a conversation or might not attempt to participate at all. Carers, family and friends are encouraged to allow the patient sufficient time to initiate and respond in conversations.

Not all people with Parkinson's disease experience difficulties with speech production. Those that do, however, suffer from weakened vocalisation, known as hypophonia, which renders the voice barely audible to the listener. Other changes result in unclear speech caused by words blending together into unintelligible sounds. The voice itself is likely to become monotone as the patient loses control over the muscles which produce the variations in pitch associated with expressing emotion. Muscular strength in the face, mouth and neck is critical not only for speech production, but also for maintaining the integrity of the airways. Weaker muscles make it difficult for people with Parkinson's to close their mouth completely and to swallow. Ineffective swallowing, or dysphagia, compromises protective airway reflexes, such as coughing, and significantly increases the risk of choking and aspiration, which are potentially life-threatening.

Early integration of a speech-language pathologist into the medical support team for people with Parkinson's is strongly recommended to reinforce the person's capacity for effective communication and to delay the onset of debilitating symptoms of the disease affecting speech, breathing, swallowing and coughing. The speech-language pathologist takes an in-depth medical history of the patient, discusses any changes in voice quality, pitch and volume and conducts acoustic analyses of the patient's voice. Initially, patients engage in individual therapy sessions which target specific voice disturbances that require intervention. Speech activities, such as enunciating frequently-used sounds, words and numbers, while using a range of volume and pitch are introduced. Referring to a voice volume meter, the patient response is measured against achievement of the decibel (dB) level indicated for each task.

To gain maximum value from speech therapy, people with PD are encouraged to commit to independent daily practice of speech exercises. The speech-language pathologist may be able to provide a complimentary booklet containing printed exercises for use during the therapy sessions and at home. As it is quite difficult for those with PD to accurately self-assess their voice volume level, they are recommended to download a voice volume meter on their smartphone for a more precise measurement. Alternatively, purpose-designed speech therapy smartphone applications, which offer a variety of practice tasks and have an integrated voice volume meter providing immediate analysis of the patient's efforts, are available and are proving to be more popular than the booklet. Both options allow unlimited attempts at each task.

The overwhelming agreement among professionals of the essential value of speech therapy to people with PD, is, unfortunately, not always reflected in the retention rates of participants in the therapy programs. Some patients who withdraw from the program report feeling bored with the repetitive voice exercises and confused about **their** relevance to everyday communication. Others, who perceive tasks involving identifying and repeating words connected to each letter of the alphabet as too simplistic and more appropriate for children than adults, are also unmotivated to continue speech therapy.

New group speech therapy treatment programs are currently being trialled to improve patient motivation and participation by incorporating meaningful activities that appeal directly to their personal interests and enhance the social aspect of natural communication. One activity which has attracted much interest involves patients with PD preparing and presenting a short talk (2-3 minutes) on a topic of their choice to fellow group members. Speech-language pathologists have observed that despite the participants initially feeling nervous, the growth in their self-confidence following their successful presentation is exceptional. Another new activity which is attracting increasing numbers of patients with PD is group singing therapy. Singing is of immense therapeutic benefit as it practises sound production focussed on clarity and volume and strengthens the muscles in the face, mouth and neck. Feedback from participants in both of these programs affirms a noticeably higher level of patient enjoyment from collaboration with others, excitement about continuing in the program and general optimism about their lives.

1. What information can be found in the first paragraph?
   A   reference to an accurate test currently available to diagnose Parkinson's disease
   B   indication of the reason for a person's lack of confidence in medical advice
   C   suggestion to delay conferring with a specialist in Parkinson's disease
   D   mention of a person's positive response to a medical opinion

2. What point is made about dopamine in paragraph 2?
   A   Medication to restore dopamine in the brain is not essential for people with Parkinson's.
   B   All patients are affected by the same Parkinson's symptoms.
   C   Dopamine loss causes characteristic signs of Parkinson's to become noticeable.
   D   Neurologists measure dopamine levels in the brain to diagnose Parkinson's.

3. The purpose of the information in paragraph 3 is to
   A   provide an explanation for the additional time needed by people with Parkinson's before speaking.
   B   infer that a person with Parkinson's prefers to avoid participation in all conversations.
   C   advise carers to continue their own conversation separately if the person with PD stops talking during the interaction.
   D   focus on the difficulties associated with reduced physical mobility.

4. In paragraph 4, what does the writer suggest about muscle strength?
   A   Changes to face and neck muscles have minimal impact on speech and swallowing.
   B   Vocalisation in PD patients with weakened muscles maintains the pitch needed to convey emotion.
   C   Reduced ability to swallow and cough effectively can result in very serious health emergencies.
   D   Hypophonia causes PD patients difficulties with hearing others.

5. According to paragraph 5, the most important objective of a speech-language pathologist in a medical support team of a person with Parkinson's is to
   A   instruct patients how to talk very loudly in every situation.
   B   prolong patient control over speech, breathing and swallowing.
   C   develop tasks that will allow patients to speak at whatever volume they choose.
   D   take a comprehensive patient history.

6 What should patients be told about speech therapy tasks?
   A It is more convenient to use the task practice booklet than a smartphone application.
   B The number of times a person can access each task in the smartphone application is restricted.
   C Patients are required to purchase a copy of the task practice booklet.
   D Routine repetition of the tasks is integral to success.

7 When the writer uses the expression 'their relevance' in paragraph 7, 'their' is referring to
   A patients who withdraw from the program.
   B the people who lead the programs.
   C tasks to identify and pronounce words connected to letters of the alphabet.
   D vocal activities that are continual and unvaried.

8 In the final paragraph, it is suggested that new approaches to group speech therapy programs
   A improve the mental wellbeing of most patients.
   B fail to inspire patients to remain in the program.
   C allow patients to become successful vocalists.
   D have an adverse effect on patients who feel anxious about 'performing' to other group members.

Write your answers here.

1	2	3	4	5	6	7	8

WRITING PRACTICE 1: LETTER OF DISCHARGE

Use the case notes to complete the writing task. You are a healthcare professional working at Green Valley Hospital. Your patient is now ready to be discharged.

TASK

- Read the case notes and use the information given to write a Letter of Discharge for your patient Mr Charles Walsh.
- Your name is Dr Jasmine Ambler.
- You are writing to the patient's general practitioner, Dr Angus Brady at Spring Hill General Practice, 15 Cherry Street, Spring Hill.
- In your letter, transform the relevant case notes into complete sentences. DO NOT USE NOTE FORM. Use a letter format.
- Assume that today's date is 5 October 2021.

CASE NOTES
GREEN VALLEY HOSPITAL
PATIENT DETAILS

NAME:	Charles David Walsh
DOB:	8 January 1948 (73 years old)
NEXT OF KIN:	Margaret Walsh (wife)
ADMISSION DATE:	4 October 2021
DISCHARGE DATE:	5 October 2021
REASON FOR ADMISSION:	Admitted via ambulance
	Fall in garden at home; warm day, lying in sun for approx. 2 hours
ASSESSMENT:	O/E pain and tenderness R chest
	Suspected fracture R ribs
SOCIAL BACKGROUND:	Retired
	Lives with wife, 2 adult children
	Non-smoker
	Non-drinker
FAMILY HISTORY:	Mother – Died post-operative MRSA infection aged 63 years
	Father – Died CVA aged 50 years
MEDICAL HISTORY:	18/02/1992 - CVA aged 44 years – full recovery
	30/06/1996 - Q fever aged 48 years
	21/10/2000 - Osteoarthritis
	03/03/2010 - Melanoma aged 62 years – excised, 3 monthly checks (indefinite referral)
	Hypertension (ongoing management)
	Eyesight ↓ cataracts removed 2016

MEDICATIONS:	Monoxidine 200mcg (1 at night)
	Perindopril/amlodipine 10mg/5mg (1 in morning)
ALLERGIES:	Pollen
PRESENTATION AND ASSESSMENT:	Right sided chest pain, worse with movement/inhalation
	Pain 10/10
	Pain non radiating, localised to right rib area
	No nausea or vomiting
	No LOC (loss of consciousness)
	Afebrile (36.9°C)
	BP 140/80 (normal)
	Pulse 85 bpm (normal)
	Respiration rate 22/min (normal)
	Alert/aware of situation
	ECG normal sinus rhythm
CHEST X-RAY:	Fracture 4th and 5th right ribs
DIAGNOSIS:	Fracture to 4th and 5th right ribs
TREATMENT AND MANAGEMENT:	Codeine/paracetamol (2 tabs orally on admission)
	IV normal saline (1L/12 hrs)
	Oxycodone (5mg, 1 tablet when required)
	Paracetamol as required
	Topical analgesic to affected area
	Physiotherapist input – deep breathing exercises hourly during waking hours - upright sitting or standing (Pt finds very painful)
	Moderate assistance required with mobility and transfers
DISCHARGE PLAN:	Recovery at home - family to assist with positioning, mobility and transfers for +/- 2 weeks
	Family to provide recliner chair, walking stick or other aid, shower chair
	Manage pain with oxycodone/naloxone (5mg/2.5mg 1 or 2 tabs twice daily); paracetamol (2 tabs as required; max 8 per day)
	Aperient once daily as needed
	Continue deep breathing exercises
	Follow up with GP in 30 days

Write your letter here.

WRITING PRACTICE 2: LETTER OF REFERRAL

Use the case notes to complete the writing task. You are the patient's general practitioner. You are referring your patient to a paediatrician.

> **TASK**
>
> - Read the case notes and use the information given to write a Letter of Referral for Harry Wheeler.
> - Your name is Dr Andrew Strickland.
> - You are writing to paediatrician Dr Marina Reyes, at Uptown Paediatrics, 92 Marshall Avenue, Central City, to request a definitive diagnosis and management of this patient.
> - In your letter, transform the relevant notes into complete sentences. DO NOT USE NOTE FORM. Use a letter format.
> - Assume that today's date is 3 November 2021.

CASE NOTES
PATIENT DETAILS

NAME:	Harry Wheeler
DOB:	23/07/2014 (age 7)
SOCIAL BACKGROUND:	Only child of married parents
	Primary school student
	Extracurricular – soccer, swimming, guitar lessons
FAMILY HISTORY:	Mother – asthma, tonsillectomy/adenoidectomy aged 10
	Father – penicillin allergy
	Maternal grandfather – OSA, migraine, asthma
	Maternal grandmother – osteoporosis
	Paternal grandfather – deceased- pancreatic cancer aged 52 years
	Paternal grandmother – coeliac
	Paternal aunts (2) – migraine, allergies (both)
	Paternal cousins - migraine
MEDICAL HISTORY:	2015 - Caesarean delivery
	2016 - ED presentation - ? gastroenteritis
	2018 - ED presentation – left otitis media – azithromycin
	2019 - Neck pain ➡ paediatric orthopaedic specialist
	2019 - X-ray - cervical spine N.A.D. (no abnormality detected)
	2020 - LRTI – prednisone, amoxicillin/clavulanic acid
	2020 - Travel sickness – medicated with OTC product
	2020 - Dermatographism – promethazine as required
	2021 - Optometrist – routine eye health check – no issues

CURRENT MEDICATIONS:	Paracetamol/ibuprofen for headaches as necessary
	OTC product for travel sickness as necessary
	Promethazine 10mg (1 at night as required)
ALLERGIES:	None known
DATE OF PRESENTATION:	19/10/2021
PRESENTING COMPLAINT:	18/10/2021 - Severe headache developed during soccer match
	On way home, eyes closed, hands over ears
	At home – drowsiness, pallor
	Pt says he felt 'very unwell'.
	Mother – 'he almost blacked out.'
	Pt slept for 3 hours and awoke without headache.
	No recent illness
	ENT/CNS exam - unremarkable
	? Viral infection
	Discussion with mother – ensure adequate sleep; limit screen time; analgesia – paracetamol or ibuprofen as required
	Instructed to re-present if headache recurs
DATE OF PRESENTATION:	03/11/2021
PRESENTING COMPLAINT:	Headaches ↑ frequency (3/14), severe
	Pt sent home from school twice
	Teacher - Pt felt 'hot'/temperature not taken; teacher contacted - confirmed no issues at school with classmates/school work
	ENT/CNS exam - normal
	Discussion with mother – family life appears normal; no sudden change to routine or relationships
	Mother ? prophylaxis for migraine; mother anxious, Pt school absences ↑
PLAN:	Requested MRI Brain – ongoing unexplained headaches/exclude intracranial pathology
	Refer to paediatrician for diagnosis and management

Write your letter here.

SPEAKING PRACTICE: MANAGING THE STRUCTURE OF DISCOURSE IN A CONSULTATION

ROLE PLAY 1

Work in pairs as healthcare professional and parent of patient. Read your role play card to familiarise yourself with the task. Take a few minutes to plan what you are going to say. You can make notes during the preparation time if you wish.

ROLE PLAY 1

ROLE A: HEALTHCARE PROFESSIONAL **SETTING: FAMILY HEALTHCARE CLINIC**

A recent blood test has confirmed that your 5-year-old patient has an iron deficiency. You are discussing treatment with the child's parent. The parent is feeling guilty about the diagnosis.

TASK

- Inform the parent that their child has a moderate iron deficiency. (The child's serum ferritin level is 11μg/L; <20μg/L in prepubescent children is diagnostic of iron deficiency.)

- Briefly explain that iron is an essential mineral and is important for a healthy immune system, which helps to fight infection.

- Enquire about the child's diet.

- Ask specifically about the quantity of red meat the child consumes.

- Explain that the child needs to eat a minimum of 3 serves of good quality red meat (beef or lamb) per week.

- Advise that dietician input is recommended if the child has trouble incorporating red meat into their diet.

- Inform the parent that the child also requires an iron supplement. Suggest that a liquid supplement would be best. The supplement should be taken every second day for 3 months.

- Suggest that the parent speaks to a pharmacist about a suitable supplement.

- Ask the parent if they have any questions.

- Reassure the parent that they have not done anything wrong. Iron deficiency is quite common in children and, with treatment, the child's ferritin levels will increase.

ROLE PLAY 1

ROLE B: PARENT OF PATIENT   SETTING: FAMILY HEALTHCARE CLINIC

Your 5-year-old child has been diagnosed with an iron deficiency. You suspect that incorporating the suggested changes into your child's diet will be difficult. You feel responsible for your child's condition and guilty that you did not recognise the problem sooner.

TASK

- When informed that your child has an iron deficiency, ask if this explains the many viruses your child has contracted recently.

- Appear pleased that you may have an explanation as to why your child has frequently been unwell recently.

- When asked about your child's diet, explain that your child eats a wide variety of mostly healthy foods. S/he particularly enjoys eating fish and avocado.

- When asked, say that your child eats very little red meat as s/he does not like the texture of meat.

- Say that you will offer more red meat at mealtimes and try very hard to encourage your child to eat more red meat. You have doubts that your efforts will be successful.

- Accept that your child may need to be referred to a dietician for advice.

- When told that your child requires supplemental iron, explain that your child will not swallow a foul-tasting liquid. Ask if it is possible for your child to have a tablet form.

- Agree to speak to a pharmacist to find the most suitable iron supplement.

- Tell the healthcare professional that you do not have any questions but you feel guilty about your child's condition and regret not becoming aware of it sooner.

ROLE PLAY 2

Work in pairs as healthcare professional and patient. Read your role play card to familiarise yourself with the task. Take a few minutes to plan what you are going to say. You can make notes during the preparation time if you wish.

ROLE PLAY 2

ROLE A: HEALTHCARE PROFESSIONAL   **SETTING: GENERAL PRACTICE CLINIC**

You have recalled a patient to discuss the findings of a recent ultrasound, which has revealed a single, relatively large gallbladder wall polyp. You are referring your patient to a specialist for management. You are informing your patient that his/her gallbladder will most likely be removed in the very near future.

TASK

- Inform your patient that the reason for the appointment is to discuss management of a large gallbladder polyp that was discovered in a recent ultrasound.

- Inform your patient that you will refer him/her to a specialist for further advice.

- Briefly explain that large gallbladder polyps pose a risk of malignancy, which needs to be managed.

- Reassure your patient and emphasise that the risk of malignancy is low.

- Inform your patient that you suspect the specialist will remove his/her gallbladder quite urgently to eliminate any risk of the polyp becoming malignant.

- Explain to your patient that he/she will most likely undergo a laparoscopic cholecystectomy, a keyhole procedure to remove the entire gallbladder.

- Reassure your patient that recovery from this procedure is usually straightforward and takes around 10 days.

- Reassure your patient that you are confident, with proper management, any risks are minimised.

ROLE PLAY 2

ROLE B: PATIENT   SETTING: GENERAL PRACTICE CLINIC

You are discussing the findings of a recent ultrasound – you have a large gallbladder wall polyp. You are being referred to a specialist for further advice. The healthcare professional is informing you that your gallbladder will probably be removed rather urgently. You are surprised and concerned by this information.

TASK

- Appear surprised upon learning about the gallbladder polyp.
- Ask why it is necessary to be referred to a specialist for a single polyp.
- Appear very concerned about the risk of potential malignancy.
- Ask what action the specialist may take.
- Appear surprised at the urgency and ask what is involved.
- Ask how long the recovery process should take.
- Emphasise that you are surprised and concerned by the urgency.

ANSWER KEY

UNIT 1 FRACTURE CARE

STUDY BOOST 1: READING AND VOCABULARY
READING 1

C   First aid for bone fractures

VOCABULARY PRACTICE 1: SENTENCE COMPLETION

0 Ensure

1   bleeding
2   still
3   Administer
4   Minimise
5   raise
6   unsure
7   straighten
8   call

READING 2

Task 1

B   Report on major contributory causes of fracture

Task 2

Questions 1-5

0   a fall, a sporting injury

1   (the) wrist, arm, elbow
2   menopause / (the) rapid decline in oestrogen levels
3   measurements of bone mineral density / bone mineral density measurements
4   calcium and vitamins D and K
5   weight-bearing exercise

Questions 6-10

6   F
7   F
8   T
9   T
10 F

VOCABULARY PRACTICE 2A: MATCHING MEANING

0	1	2	3	4	5	6	7	8	9	10
I	F	D	H	J	C	B	G	K	A	E

VOCABULARY PRACTICE 2B: COMPLETE THE SENTENCE

0 sedentary
1 adolescence / fragile
2 prone to
3 reserves / depletes / mineral
4 associated with
5 deficiency / adversely / significant

READING 3

0 C
1 B
2 C
3 A
4 B
5 C
6 B

VOCABULARY PRACTICE 3: COMPLETE THE SENTENCE

0 B
1 C
2 A
3 C
4 B
5 A
6 C

STUDY BOOST 2: SPEAKING

SPEAKING PRACTICE 1: MULTIPLE CHOICE

0 B
1 A
2 B
3 B
4 A
5 A
6 B
7 B
8 B
9 B
10 A

UNIT 2   ALLERGY SYMPTOM RELIEF

STUDY BOOST 1: READING AND VOCABULARY

READING 1

Task 1

B   A specific allergen commonly found indoors

Task 2

0   T
1   F
2   T
3   T
4   F
5   F
6   F
7   T
8   T

VOCABULARY PRACTICE 1: MATCHING MEANING

0	1	2	3	4	5	6	7	8	9	10
B	J	D	F	A	G	I	C	E	K	H

READING 2

0   A
1   B
2   C
3   B
4   A
5   B

VOCABULARY PRACTICE 2: WORD FORMS

0   B
1   B
2   A
3   C
4   C
5   A

READING 3

0   B
1   C
2   A
3   B
4   C
5   A

STUDY BOOST 2: WRITING
WRITING PRACTICE 1: UNDERSTANDING AND USING CAPITAL LETTERS

0 <u>**Thank you for seeing Sean Mulrooney in regard to his recent diagnosis of Parkinson's disease.**</u>

1 **D**ear **D**r **L**arkham

2 **P**lease present to the admissions desk at **C**ityside **H**ospital at 0800 on **F**riday, **A**ugust 12.

3 **M**r **S**ingh takes **N**asonex and **Z**yrtec as needed.

4 **M**rs **M**artin has been advised to take paracetamol (a maximum of 8 per day) to manage pain. **H**er preference is to take **P**anadol rather than a generic brand.

5 **L**ouisa **S**haw was born in **B**oston, **M**assachusetts in **J**uly 1978.

6 **Y**ours sincerely

   Dr **A**my **L**iu

7 **S**he is from **L**ismore which is in **C**ounty **W**aterford in **I**reland.

8 **T**he faecal test returned a positive result for **G**iardia intestinalis and **I** have organised repeat testing following treatment with **F**lagyl, 400mg 3 times daily for 7 days.

9 **O**cean **V**iew **R**espite **C**are

   15 **K**ennedy **T**errace

   Beach **B**ay

   New **S**outh **W**ales

10 **T**he most recent outbreak of **E**bola began in the **D**emocratic **R**epublic of **C**ongo in **A**ugust.

11 **M**r **S**ong is from **S**outh **K**orea and requires an interpreter as he does not speak **E**nglish.

12 **W**e note from our records that you are now due for your routine dental examination.

Writing Practice 2: Error correction

00 ✔

0 **Easy Steps Podiatry**

1 blood pressure

2 disease

3 physiotherapist

4 Hill

5 ibuprofen

6 ✔

7 allergic rhinitis

8 ambulance

9 spleen

10 laser eye surgery

11 Hospital

12 ✔

WRITING PRACTICE 3: USING CAPITAL LETTERS IN MEDICAL CORRESPONDENCE

Letter 1

Dr Bruno Martini

Valley Allergy Specialists

Suite 155, Greenway House

56 Market Street

Paddington

____ July 20___

Dear **B**runo

Re: **D**ario **D**i **D**io, aged 50

Thank you for seeing **M**r **D**ario **D**i **D**io, aged 50 years, for allergy testing and management of his ongoing symptoms.

Mr **D**i **D**io has had intermittent nausea, headaches and fatigue for 2 years. **T**he onset of symptoms occurred after an episode of gastroenteritis as a result of a **H**elicobacter pylori infection.

I have performed a range of investigations, including a recent urea breath test to exclude **H**. pylori recurrence, the results of which were negative. **C**opies are attached.

I have no other investigations planned at this time. **A**s **I** have not found a clear pathology to target for treatment, **I** would be grateful for your specialist advice.

Thank you for your care and management.

Yours sincerely

Dr **A**lessio **G**reco

Letter 2

Dr Alessio Greco
Family Medical Practice
97 Mulberry Terrace
Sunnyside

____ July 20___

Dear Alessio

Re: Mr Dario Di Dio

Dario Di Dio attended an appointment on May 19 to undergo allergy testing.

A skin prick test was used to test 32 potential allergens. Mr Di Dio tested positive to the dust mite allergen.

The recommended treatment is nasal rinsing with saline once per week using a commercially available product, an intranasal corticosteroid available over-the-counter, 2 sprays in each nostril, once per day, and dust mite protectors on all bedding including the mattress. (We recommend Allergex brand.)

If his symptoms fail to resolve, I recommend that Mr Di Dio should return to us for immunotherapy. This will involve one injection of a solution containing the dust mite allergen every month for 5 years.

I have also referred Mr Di Dio to dietician Giorgia Chiari for advice on commencing an elimination diet as his symptoms are also suggestive of a food chemical intolerance.

Thank you for referring this patient to Valley Allergy Specialists.

Yours sincerely

Dr Bruno Martini

UNIT 3 DIABETES MANAGEMENT

STUDY BOOST 1: READING AND VOCABULARY
READING 1

0 C
1 A
2 B
3 B
4 C
5 A
6 C

VOCABULARY PRACTICE 1A: MATCHING MEANING

0	1	2	3	4	5	6	7	8	9	10
F	K	G	E	J	D	C	A	I	H	B

VOCABULARY PRACTICE 1B: COMPLETE THE SENTENCE

0 consistent
1 Subsequent
2 screening
3 compensate
4 blurry
5 life-threatening

READING 2

0 C
1 B
2 A
3 C
4 B
5 A

VOCABULARY PRACTICE 2: WORD FORMS

0 B interpretation
1 C calibrated
2 A implant
3 C Technological
4 B Fluctuating
5 A depression

READING 3

0	1	2	3	4	5	6	7	8	9	10
E	G	J	K	I	B	H	D	A	F	C

VOCABULARY PRACTICE 3: WORD FORMATION

0 complication
1 prolonged
2 swelling
3 retention
4 frequently

5 nauseous
6 filtration / filtering
7 assessed
8 Progression
9 failure
10 weight

STUDY BOOST 2: SPEAKING

SPEAKING PRACTICE 1: CHOOSE THE APPROPRIATE RESPONSE

0 D
1 A
2 F
3 J
4 I
5 K
6 C
7 B
8 G
9 H
10 E

UNIT 4   FOCUS ON COMMON ERRORS 1: SPELLING

STUDY BOOST 1: READING AND VOCABULARY

Task 1

00	0	1	2	3	4	5	6	7	8	9	10
G	K	L	F	I	H	C	J	E	A	B	D

STUDY BOOST 2

Task 2

This is a sample template. Answers for this task will vary for each person.

Personal common error register

Base word	Meaning	Noun form	Verb form	Adjective form	Adverb form	Plural form

WRITING PRACTICE 1: SPOT THE ERROR

COLUMN A: WORDS SPELLED CORRECTLY IN BOX ✔	COLUMN B: REWRITE INCORRECTLY SPELLED WORDS IN BOX USING CORRECT SPELLING.
(0) beginning	(00) importance
reference	re**comm**endation
attendance	artifici**a**l
prescribe	a**d**justment
inhibitor	a**ss**ociation
specialize (US) specialise (GB)	va**cc**inate
strategy	resu**s**citate
subscription	acco**mm**odation
maintenance	refe**rr**ing
stability	infla**mm**ation
mobilise (British) mobilize (US)	occurr**e**nce
sustenance	u**n**necessary
negligent	

WRITING PRACTICE 2: ERROR CORRECTION

Letter 1 – Letter of Referral from dentist to endodontist

0   presented
1   experiencing
2   ✔
3   management
4   likelihood
5   integrity
6   paracetamol
7   ✔
8   infection
9   assessment
10 ✔
11 hesitate
12 sincerely

Letter 2 - Letter from endodontist to dentist

13 referring
14 ✔
15 severe
16 advised
17 ✔
18 precautionary
19 ✔
20 arrange
21 sincerely

UNIT 5 CONSOLIDATION 1 (UNITS 1-4)

READING PRACTICE

Questions 1-8

0	1	2	3	4	5	6	7	8
A	C	B	D	B	D	A	B	C

Questions 9-15

9 changes to vision or severe headache which does not respond to pain relief

10 (on average) between 3-6 weeks

11 to check/measure reduced cartilage space in these joints

12 Choose 2 from these options:
   isolation/withdrawal from family and friends
   behavioural differences, including mood swings
   poor appetite
   interrupted sleep patterns
   depression

13 (try) an elimination diet

14 mornings/ in the morning

15 (an) elevated level of inflammation

Questions 16-20

16 to manage/of managing/ to control/of controlling/ to adapt to/of adapting to

17 risk of heart

18 inflammatory heat

19 prevent/reduce the risk of severe damage

20 5-20

WRITING PRACTICE 1: ERROR CORRECTION (CAPITAL LETTERS)

Letter 1: Referral from general practitioner (GP) to physiotherapist

00 Dylan

0 ✔

1 osteoarthritis

2 She

3 ✔

4 ✔

5 physiotherapist

6 Moxicam

7 ✔

8 ✔

9 sincerely

10 Dr

WRITING PRACTICE 2: ERROR CORRECTION (SPELLING)

Letter 2: Letter from physiotherapist to general practitioner (GP)

00 ✔
0 referring
1 palpation
2 ✔
3 cartilage
4 ✔
5 menisci
6 ✔
7 sustained
8 ✔
9 weight
10 separate
11 symptoms
12 recommended
13 ✔
14 ✔
15 advised
16 compliance
17 information
18 sincerely

UNIT 6   GASTROINTESTINAL INVESTIGATIONS

STUDY BOOST 1: READING AND VOCABULARY

READING 1

Task 1

Text A:	iii)	FOOD CHEMICAL ELIMINATION PLAN
Text B:	ii)	CANINE INFECTIOUS AGENTS SCREENING
Text C:	i)	ULTRASOUND OF UPPER ABDOMEN
Text D:	iv)	PATHOLOGY TEST RESULTS

Task 2

Questions 1-6

0	1	2	3	4	5	6
A	D	C	B	A	C	B

Questions 7-10

7 3 consecutive days (without symptoms)
8 (the) pancreas
9 (acute) diarrhoea and vomiting
10 headaches, fatigue, nausea, diarrhoea

Questions 11-15

11 antibiotic (containing carboxypenicillins including ticarcillin)
12 genetic variants
13 Choose any 3 - bowel cancer/coeliac disease/diverticulitis/NSAID ulceration/chronic inflammation
14 12
15 50mg/kg

VOCABULARY PRACTICE 1A: MATCHING MEANING

0	1	2	3	4	5	6	7	8	9	10
D	K	H	F	G	J	I	B	E	A	C

VOCABULARY PRACTICE 1B: COMPLETE THE SENTENCE

0 remission
1 methodology
2 Echogenic
3 validated
4 elevated
5 eliminate, reaction
6 conclusive
7 ulceration

READING 2

0 T
1 T
2 F
3 F
4 F
5 T

VOCABULARY PRACTICE 2: ERROR CORRECTION

00 ✔
0 about
1 ✔
2 of
3 in
4 ✔
5 ✔
6 ✔
7 to
8 ✔

READING 3

0	1	2	3	4	5	6	7	8
A	F	C	I	E	D	G	B	H

VOCABULARY PRACTICE 3: WORD FORMATION

0 commonly
1 controlled
2 Perforation
3 uncommon
4 infection
5 inhalation
6 procedure
7 unstable
8 sedation/sedative
9 difficulty/difficulties
10 abdominal

STUDY BOOST 2: WRITING

WRITING PRACTICE 1

Headings

A ADDRESS
B DATE
C OPENING SALUTATION
D REFERENCE TO WHOM OR WHAT THE LETTER IS ABOUT
E INTRODUCTION
F BODY - INVESTIGATIONS PERFORMED
G BODY – TREATMENT
H CONCLUSION
I COMPLIMENTARY CLOSE

WRITING PRACTICE 2

0	1	2	3	4	5	6	7	8	9
I	H	A	E	H	F	D	E	G	E

WRITING PRACTICE 3

0	1	2	3	4	5	6	7	8	9
B	F	D	I	A	J	G	H	C	E

UNIT 7 INFECTION PREVENTION AND CONTROL

STUDY BOOST 1: READING AND VOCABULARY

READING 1

0 B
1 C
2 A
3 B
4 C
5 B
6 B

VOCABULARY PRACTICE 1A: MATCHING REFERENCE PRONOUNS

0	1	2	3	4	5	6
E	A	F	B	C	G	D

VOCABULARY PRACTICE 1B: WORD FORMS

0	1	2	3	4	5	6	7	8	9	10
C	B	A	C	A	C	B	C	A	C	B

READING 2

1	2	3	4	5	6	7	8
B	C	A	D	C	A	D	B

VOCABULARY PRACTICE 2: SENTENCE COMPLETION

0	1	2	3	4	5	6	7	8
B	G	A	C	D	F	E	I	H

READING 3: COMPLETE THE SENTENCE

0	1	2	3	4	5	6	7	8	9	10
C	E	G	J	B	I	A	F	K	H	D

STUDY BOOST 2: SPEAKING

SPEAKING PRACTICE 1A: COMPLETE THE SENTENCE

0 C because
1 A due to
2 C to summarise
3 B Having said that
4 B especially
5 C unlike
6 A First of all
7 B because
8 B for example
9 C Incidentally
10 A However

SPEAKING PRACTICE 1B: MULTIPLE CHOICE CLOZE

0 C First
1 B and
2 C Alternatively
3 A therefore
4 B whereas
5 C unfortunately
6 A Fortunately
7 C Incidentally
8 B such as
9 A All the same
10 C Above all

UNIT 8   MEDICAL EMERGENCIES

STUDY BOOST 1: READING AND VOCABULARY

READING 1

0	1	2	3	4	5	6
B	B	A	C	C	B	A

VOCABULARY PRACTICE 1A: MATCHING MEANING

0	1	2	3	4	5	6	7	8	9	10
D	C	J	I	K	H	A	G	B	F	E

VOCABULARY PRACTICE 1B: SENTENCE COMPLETION

0	1	2	3	4	5	6	7	8	9	10	11	12
H	A	J	B	I	C	D	M	G	F	K	L	E

READING 2
QUESTIONS 1-6

0	1	2	3	4	5	6
F	D	E	B	A	C	E

QUESTIONS 7-10

7 ≤90 minutes
8 wrist and groin
9 organisation and storage of cosmetics in coloured boxes
10 real world challenges e.g. full lifts, interruptions

QUESTIONS 11-15

11	12	13	14	15
B	C	C	B	A

VOCABULARY PRACTICE 2A: MATCHING REFERENCE PRONOUNS

Example Text B	A	B	C	D	E	F
vii	iii	v	iv	i	vi	ii

VOCABULARY PRACTICE 2B: WORD FORMS

0	1	2	3	4	5	6	7	8	9	10
A	B	A	C	B	C	C	B	A	C	A

READING 3: COMPLETE THE SENTENCE

0	1	2	3	4	5	6	7	8	9	10
C	J	D	H	K	E	B	A	G	I	F

STUDY BOOST 2: WRITING

WRITING PRACTICE 1: SELECTING RELEVANT CASE NOTES

1 Dr Pamela Smith
2 Letter of Discharge – transferring to a rehabilitation facility/Letter of Transfer

RELEVANT – INCLUDE	NOT RELEVANT – DO NOT INCLUDE
Patient's name – James Adams AGE: 44 years old DOB: 4 April 1977 ADMISSION DATE: 16 May 2021 DISCHARGE DATE: 20 May 2021 REASON FOR ADMISSION: ? CVA DIAGNOSIS: CVA caused by possible vasospasm SOCIAL BACKGROUND: works full time – personal trainer PRESENTATION AND ASSESSMENT: right-sided weakness, esp. hand, slurred speech, sharp head pain, LOC approx. 30 secs, slightly confused, no pain, BP, pulse, temperature, admit for obs MRI/CT HEAD: unremarkable TREATMENT AND MANAGEMENT: assisted ++ with ADLs, aspirin – 81mg daily, physiotherapy – daily – restore hand function and regain balance ➜ slow improvement ➜ to rehab, 5-day program and reassess, speech therapy – daily – restore speech – good progress, monitored 4 days, mobile with supervision DISCHARGE PLAN: Discharge ➜ rehabilitation centre – hand function and balance, writing practice ++, aspirin – 81mg daily, review on discharge from rehab, discussion – Pt keen to return to full function for work	*Patient's next of kin – Michael Adams* SOCIAL BACKGROUND: lives alone, former smoker, minimal alcohol FAMILY HISTORY: mother – angina, father – deceased MI aged 52 years MEDICAL HISTORY: nil significant MEDICATIONS: none recorded ALLERGIES: none known PRESENTATION AND ASSESSMENT: admitted via ambulance, O² therapy given TREATMENT AND MANAGEMENT: BP 130/65 on discharge, pulse 80 bpm on discharge

WRITING PRACTICE 2: COMPLETE THE SENTENCE

0 the
1 on
2 a
3 due to
4 has had
5 and
6 her
7 were
8 at
9 she
10 which
11 has been
12 however

WRITING PRACTICE 3: COMPLETE THE SENTENCE

00 whom
0 biliary colic
1 indigestion
2 vomiting
3 10 hours
4 over-the-counter
5 appetite
6 right upper quadrant
7 presented to
8 which
9 codeine/paracetamol
10 trial/be trialling
11 gastro-oesophageal reflux
12 they

WRITING PRACTICE 4: SELECTING AND TRANSFORMING CASE NOTES

0	C	after collapsing at home
1	H	for approximately 2 minutes
2	S	to his left ear
3	L	there was no indication
4	B	were both normal
5	P	was largely unremarkable
6	R	is also a possibility
7	D	and dressed with
8	F	was observed
9	N	abnormality was detected
10	A	within 12 hours
11	J	in the care of his wife
12	G	is to increase
13	K	the dressing to
14	Q	for review of hypertension
15	M	follow-up appointment

WRITING EXTENSION TASK

(Sample Answer from Case Notes in Writing Practice 1)

Dr Pamela Smith

76 West Avenue

Springfield

20 May 2021

Dear Dr Smith

Re: Mr James Adams 04/04/1977

Mr Adams is being admitted to your care as further therapy is indicated to restore hand and balance function following a cerebrovascular accident.

Mr Adams presented to the emergency department at Cannonvale Hospital on 16/5/21, having experienced sharp head pain and loss of consciousness for approximately 30 seconds. On examination, he had right sided weakness, temporary slight confusion and slurred speech. His blood pressure and pulse were elevated and his temperature was normal. No pain was reported. MRI and CT of the brain were unremarkable. He was admitted for further observation.

The diagnosis was cerebrovascular accident with vasospasm as the possible cause.

He required moderate assistance with ADLs and undertook daily physiotherapy to restore function to hand and balance with limited results. As Mr Adams works as a personal trainer, he is keen to return to full physical function. In particular, he needs to continue to practise writing. There was noticeable improvement in speech after 4 days of speech therapy.

He was commenced on aspirin, 81mg daily, to be reviewed prior to discharge from your care.

Please do not hesitate to contact me should you require further details.

Yours sincerely

Dr Jacqueline Stratton

UNIT 9 FOCUS ON COMMON ERRORS 2: FORMAL AND INFORMAL LANGUAGE

STUDY BOOST 1

Task 1

0	1	2	3	4	5	6
F	D	E	B	G	C	A

STUDY BOOST 2

Task 2

0	1	2	3	4	5	6	7	8	9	10	11	12
L	S	J	Z	X	Q	T	W	R	C	V	A	F

13	14	15	16	17	18	19	20	21	22	23	24	25
U	N	G	Y	E	I	D	M	B	O	P	H	K

WRITING PRACTICE: SENTENCE TRANSFORMATION

Part 1

00 is required to

1 will be postponed/is going to be postponed
2 becoming/getting/being/ infected with
3 are investigating
4 (which is) absorbed by
5 was rescheduled to/for an

Part 2

0 's/ is about how

6 weeks to get over a
7 flared up
8 puffed up
9 couldn't / could not put up with
10 throwing up

SPEAKING PRACTICE: MULTIPLE CHOICE

0	1	2	3	4	5	6	7	8	9	10
B	A	B	B	A	B	A	B	B	A	B

Q	A= formal B= informal	Additional information to support answers in context
0	B	**Julio and Su Jin are colleagues who know each other well. It is appropriate for them to be speaking informally 'off duty' to each other about their social plans**
1	A	The patient is elderly and should be addressed with respect. The instructions use standard English, are clear and will be understood by the patient.
2	B	The nurse sets a reassuring, trusting tone, including using her first name in the introduction so that patients will feel more comfortable.
3	B	Lymphoma care nurse, Donna, understands the patient is confused and worried. She reassures the patient and uses simplified language, rather than official medical terms, to explain the treatment plan to the patient.
4	A	This is a formal induction. It's important to give all essential information in a clear and logical way, using official terminology e.g. donning and doffing gloves.
5	B	The patient is an 8-year-old child who is feeling anxious. The nurse uses direct, age-appropriate language that is comprehensible and reassuring to the patient.
6	A	This is a formal presentation by a senior staff member to student trainees. It is important to deliver all essential information in a logical, clear manner.
7	B	The nurse is providing the carer with a detailed list of instructions using clear accessible language. The nurse reassures the carer that he has ongoing access to all the instructions in the discharge pack.
8	B	The hand therapist uses age-appropriate language to explain the treatment to the child and to reduce the child's anxiety.
9	A	This is a formal presentation about a medical procedure given to a group of Junior Residents. The information must be explicit, accurate and use appropriate medical terminology.
10	B	The nurse is using language that is comprehensible to the patient to clarify the situation and reassure the patient who is worried about an eye injury.

UNIT 10 CONSOLIDATION 2 ANSWER KEY

READING PRACTICE

Questions 1-8

1	2	3	4	5	6	7	8
B	C	A	C	B	D	D	A

WRITING PRACTICE 1: SAMPLE ANSWER-LETTER OF DISCHARGE

Dr Angus Brady

Spring Hill General Practice

15 Cherry Street

Spring Hill

5 October 2021

Dear Dr Dermott

Re: Mr Charles David Walsh (aged 72)

Mr Walsh was admitted to Green Valley Hospital via ambulance on 4 October (year) with suspected fracture to right ribs following a fall in his garden. He presented with severe pain (10/10) to the right chest which was aggravated by movement of the upper body.

The diagnosis was fracture to the right 4th and 5th ribs.

Pain and tenderness to the right chest, especially on inhaling were noted on examination. Blood pressure was 140/80 and temperature, pulse and respiration rates were unremarkable. There was no loss of consciousness. The patient was alert and aware of the situation. An ECG was conducted as a precaution and no abnormality was detected. X-ray confirmed fracture to right 4th and 5th ribs.

Codeine/paracetamol was administered immediately for pain relief (2 tablets, orally) upon arrival at hospital. Normal saline was administered intravenously (1 litre over 12 hours) to prevent dehydration. Moderate assistance was required with mobility and transfers.

A physiotherapist assessed Mr Walsh and prescribed deep breathing exercises which he finds very painful. He is to continue with these deep breathing exercises at home (hourly when awake) in an upright sitting or standing position to improve lung function and prevent complications.

Pain is being managed with oxycodone/naloxone (5mg, 1 to 2 tablets 6 hourly) and paracetamol (500mg x 2, 6 hourly). An aperient can be taken once daily as needed.

Mr Walsh will continue to recover at home with the support of his family. He will require assistance with mobility and positioning for approximately 2 weeks. His family will provide a recliner chair, walking stick and shower chair for use at home.

He is to follow up with you in approximately one month.

Please contact me if you have any queries.

Yours sincerely,

Dr Jasmine Ambler

WRITING PRACTICE 2: SAMPLE ANSWER-LETTER OF REFERRAL

Dr Marina Reyes
Uptown Paediatrics
92 Marshall Ave
Central City

3 November 2021

Dear Dr Reyes

Re: Harry Wheeler

Thank you for seeing Harry Wheeler, aged 7 years, who presented today with a recent history of severe headaches. I am referring Harry to you for further investigation and management.

Harry's first headache developed suddenly during a game of soccer on 18/10/21. He had been in good health until this point. He describes being sensitive to light and sound at the time of the headache and feeling 'very unwell'. His mother reported drowsiness and pallor. The headache resolved with sleep.

Harry has experienced several severe headaches since, which have disrupted his attendance at school. I prescribed paracetamol and ibuprofen but the patient says that the pain is not well controlled. Harry's mother is anxious about his increasing number of school absences and is hopeful that prophylactic treatment may be appropriate for him.

There is no prior history of headaches and a recent eye examination revealed no issues. I performed two ENT and CNS examinations and both were unremarkable. There appear to be no school-related problems or conflict with peers or within the family group. I note there is a strong family history of migraine.

I have requested MRI to exclude intracranial pathology, the results of which I will forward to you when they become available.

I would be grateful if you could provide a definitive diagnosis for this patient. Please do not hesitate to contact me if you require further information.

Yours sincerely,

Dr Andrew Strickland

www.ingramcontent.com/pod-product-compliance
Lightning Source LLC
Chambersburg PA
CBHW061536010526
44107CB00066B/2878